# Nursing Fundamentals I & II

***Subcourses MD0905 & MD0906***

***Edition 100***

AF859548

# Nursing Fundamentals I & II

***Subcourses MD0905 & MD0906***

***Edition 100***

**Nursing Fundamentals I & II: Subcourses MD0905 & MD0906, Edition 100**



PharmaLogika, Inc.
PO Box 461
Willow Springs, NC 27592

www.pharmalogika.com

PharmaLogika Books is an imprint of PharmaLogika, Inc. PharmaLogika and its logos are trademarks of PharmaLogika, Inc. All other trademarks used herein are the properties of their respective owners and are used for identification purposes only.



*Author / Editor*: Mindy J. Allport-Settle

Published by PharmaLogika, Inc.

Printed in the United States of America.

ISBN 1-9372580-1-7
ISBN-13 978-1-937258-01-6

# Contents

## Nursing Fundamentals II

# Overview

## About this Book

The United States Army is recognized internationally as the standard for complete, efficient and effective adult education. The Army has a tradition of pioneering training systems (including computer based training) that then transition into the corporate sector.

This manual has been continuously tested and updated to successfully educate every member of the modern United States Army. The needs of the instructor, the student, and the Army are perfectly balanced. This is the model all educators strive to follow when developing and delivering training programs.

### Included Documents and Features

#### Nursing Fundamentals I

1. Patient Relations
    - Section I. Basic Human Needs and Principles of Health
    - Section II. Communication Skills
    - Section III. Reaction to Stress and Hospitalization
    - Section IV. Transcultural Factors Influencing Nursing Care
2. The Adult Patient Care Unit
3. Advanced Principles of Patient Hygiene
4. Body Mechanics
    - Section I. Techniques of Body Mechanics
    - Section II. Positioning and Ambulating the Adult Patient
5. Active and Passive Range of Motion Exercises
6. Environmental Health and the Practical Nurse

#### Nursing Fundamentals II

1. Assisting with the Physical Examination

# Introduction

As a member of the Army Nurse Corps, your role as an Army Officer will afford you the chance to care for your patients in a variety of settings. Army Nurses have autonomy to practice nursing in a way that is unmatched by civilian health care facilities. Your professional judgment will be the driving force behind leading your nursing team to provide full spectrum patient care.

The Army Nurse Corps believes in a holistic nursing philosophy. You'll identify and organize multi disciplinary resources for patients and their families to help them with inpatient, outpatient and home care. You'll be able to understand the special concerns and needs of your Soldier patients because you're also a Soldier, which allows you to better serve them. Identifying with your fellow Soldiers is essential to providing effective health care. Explore your options in the Army Nurse Corps below.

## *History of the Army Nurse Corps*

The United States Army Nurse Corps (NC) was formally established by the U.S. Congress in 1901. It is one of the six medical Special Branches (or "Corps") of officers which along with medical enlisted soldiers comprise the Army Medical Department (AMEDD).

The NC is the nursing service for the U.S. Army and provides qualified nursing staff in support of the Department of Defense medical plans. This NC is composed entirely of registered nurses (RNs).

### Ready, Caring, Proud

Since 1901, Army nurses have demonstrated again and again their total commitment to the highest standards of military nursing excellence. Both men and women have served as Army nurses since 1775, but the Army Nurse Corps did not become a part of the Army Medical Department until 1901. The distinguished contributions of female contract nurses during and following the

1898 Spanish American War became the justification and demonstrated the need for a permanent female nurse corps.[1]

When the United States entered World War I in 1917, there were only 4,093 nurses on active duty. By November 1918, there were 21,460 Army nurses, with 10,000 serving overseas. During the war, nurses served primarily in base, evacuation, and mobile surgical hospitals in the United States, France, Hawaii, Puerto Rico, and the Philippines. They also provided care on hospital trains in France and transport ships carrying wounded home across the Atlantic. Approximately 270 nurses lost their lives in the conflict.

When the United States entered World War II, fewer than 7,000 nurses were on active duty. By 1945, more than 57,000 Army Nurses were assigned to hospital ships and trains, flying ambulances, field hospitals, evacuation stations, and general hospitals at home and overseas. In Europe, Army nurses assisted in developing the concept of recovery wards for immediate postoperative nursing care. Military nursing gained a greater understanding of the process of shock, blood replacement, and resuscitation. Air evacuation from the combat zone by fixed wing aircraft brought patients to definitive treatment quickly. Army flight nurses helped to establish the incredible record of only five deaths in flight per 100,000 patients.

Nurses endured hardships caring for their patients. In May 1942, with the fall of Corregidor in the Philippines, 67 Army nurses became Japanese prisoners of war. During the thirty seven month captivity, the women endured primitive conditions and starvation rations, yet they continued to care for the ill and injured in the internment hospital. On Anzio, nurses dug their foxholes outside their tents and cared for patients under German shellfire. Their example bolstered the spirits of the soldiers who shared the same tough experience. By war's end, 215 brave nurses died for their country.

Army nurses once again played a major role in support of combat troops when President Truman ordered United States forces into Korea in June, 1950. Army nurses cared for combat troops during the landing on Inchon; the advance across the 38th parallel into North Korea; the amphibious landing on the east coast of Korea; the drive toward the Yalu River; and the retreat to the 38th parallel. Throughout the Korean War, 540 Army nurses served on the embattled peninsula.

Mobility and increased patient acuity characterized service in Vietnam. Evacuation by helicopter brought wounded to medical units located within

---

[1] Army Nurse Corps Historical Collection documents summarized by MAJ Debora Cox, Past ANC Historian (1 August 2001). Available on the U.S. Army website at: http://history.amedd.army.mil/ANCWebsite/about.html

minutes flying time of the battlefield. The UH 1H helicopter ambulance, nicknamed the "Dustoff," not only transported patient from battle locations fifty percent faster than in Korea, but also provided triage and resuscitative services for casualties. Trauma care specialization, as well as shock/trauma units, developed from this experience. The "chain of evacuation" from Vietnam was extraordinary. A soldier could be wounded on the battlefield one day and two days later be in an Army hospital in the continental United States. In Vietnam, of the nearly 5,000 Army Nurses who served in forty four hospitals, eight women made the ultimate sacrifice for their nation.

During Operation Desert Storm, approximately 2,200 nurses served in forty four hospitals. Two of every three nurses in the Arabian Gulf were from the Army National Guard or Army Reserves. This was the first major conflict that DEPMEDS, Deployable Medical Systems, were used. Another unique feature was that Army hospital staff coexisted with host nation personnel in fixed facilities forming joint national professional organizations. Before, during, and after the 100 hour ground war, U.S. forces sustained a disease and non battle injury rate that was the lowest ever recorded in a conflict.

Recent years have seen Army nurses active throughout the world both in armed conflicts and humanitarian endeavors. In 1983, they supported combat troops in Grenada; in 1989 in Panama; and in 1991 in the Middle East. Since December 1995, Army nurses have been deployed with medical units in support of NATO alliance troops in Haiti, Bosnia, Herzegovina and Kosovo. Nurses have continued to serve proudly during relief efforts following natural disasters such as Hurricane Mitch in 1998. Today, the legacy of these military nurses lives on. Currently, Army nurses serve throughout the world in support of multiple military and humanitarian actions in support of the Global War On Terrorism.

The Corps' recent professional evolution reflects not only the requirement of a transformational Army, but also its expanded roles in support of the health care needs of the nation. Army nurses compete with other members of the Army Medical Department for command positions. For example, our current Chief, Major General Gale S. Pollock, is the first Army Nurse Corps Chief to be appointed a 2 star general. She is also the Commanding General of Tripler Amy Medical Center, Pacific Regional Medical Command, United States Army Pacific Surgeon and Lead Agent TRICARE Pacific Honolulu, Hawaii.

Throughout its history, the Army Nurse Corps has earned the deep respect and gratitude of the American people because of its dedication to providing the best possible care to our soldiers and their families while serving our country in war and peace. Army nurses have unselfishly come to the aid of victims of disaster and disease throughout the world. Over time, the mission has grown broader, yet there has been one constant the devotion of the individual nurse in providing excellent nursing care.

Today, as our soldiers stand on point for our nation, defending freedom across the globe, they can rest assured, should they get wounded or ill, an Army nurse will be by their side during their hour of need. Because any time our nation calls: "Ready, Caring, and Proud," Army nurses always respond.

## *Army Nurse Corps Campaign Plan*

### Situation

The nation's nursing shortage continues to have the potential to negatively impact the quality and safety of patient care both in civilian and military medical treatment facilities (MTF). Insufficient Army nursing capacity and in some cases low density specialties can threaten the viability of current and future AMEDD missions.[2]

The use of different nursing care delivery models in MTFs increases practice variance, limits the capability to codify evidence based nursing practice and causes imbalanced nursing workload to workforce ratios across the AMEDD. An inability to offer innovative, flexible career programs that promote nurse retention further decrements the steadystate workforce that is needed for workforce optimization. An irrelevant long range leader succession plan and appropriate force structure precludes optimization of key leader knowledge and skills required for organizational traction and momentum. No corporate, cohesive nurse training blueprint exists that leverages human capital asymmetric advantages such as junior nurses' capabilities to innovate in complex, uncertain environments that can mitigate gaps in technology and nursing capacity. The sustained increased demand for Army nurses is beginning to exceed the sustainable supply. As a result, Army nursing's ability to respond proactively to new and different contingencies is decreasing. Twenty first century persistent conflicts demand fullspectrum Army nurses who are versatile in their ability to accomplish a broad range of tasks and agile thinkers who can exploit opportunities in complex environments.

Hospital based Army Nurse Corps' medical occupational specialties and additional skill identifiers were developed for a hospital based environment in an era where the Army was downsizing. New MOS/ASI's are required to provide the right expeditionary and interoperable capability in support of the strength of our Nation: America's Army. Emerging global trends impacting the

---

[2] Available for download from the U.S. Army website ar: http://armynursecorps.amedd.army.mil/campaign/campaignplanonwebpagemarch09.pdf

Army demand an analysis and optimization of the Army Nurse Corps force horizon.

## Key Assumptions

- The nursing shortage is a looming public health crisis that has the potential to erode access to and quality of military health care.
- Nurses are critical to meeting the increasing healthcare needs of vulnerable populations.
- Competitive edge strategies will attract and retain qualified nurses and nurse candidates from an increasingly diverse population.
- Nurses have a responsibility to impact needed changes in healthcare delivery systems and models of care.
- Nurses function as partners in an interdisciplinary healthcare delivery system.
- Current and future military healthcare delivery systems demand predictive models that delineate required nursing capacities and capabilities.
- Current and future changes in nursing workload texture demand measurement systems that capture workload quality and quantity; promote nurse staffing models and improve nursing care performance improvement.

## Purpose

This Army Nurse Corps Campaign Plan establishes priorities for the Corps and codifies campaign planning as the systematic process for blueprinting the future.

Major improvements in agility often require new work systems, simplification of work processes, or an ability to rapidly change direction towards improvement. Subsequently, a major long term investment associated with nursing care excellence is the investment in creating and sustaining an assessment system focused on outcomes.

The priorities drive strategic planning and are conducted to nest with the AMEDD's and Army's mission and vision. These priorities include measures of effectiveness ("are we doing the right things") and measures of performance ("are we doing things right") that indicate when the priority has been accomplished and becomes sustainable. On receipt of this Plan, all Action

Officers will form a process action team to develop their strategy and way ahead. The strategy must include resources required, designated benchmarks (date or condition), priority or enabling tasks identified, and a timeline for execution.

The plan is evaluated yearly by the ANC Executive Board and approved by the Chief, AN. The Deputy Chief, AN evaluates progress on the plan monthly and reports accordingly to the Chief, AN. Transparency is optimum and the Chief AN will provide updates to DSG, TSG and Congress as often as requested.

An effective Army Nurse Corps depends on the continuous measurement and analysis of performance. Subsequently, campaign planning occurs yearly to evaluate performance, codify and internalize best practices and transform key work processes and systems to achieve performance excellence.

## Army Nurse Corps Campaign Plan Mission and End State

### A. Mission

#### *Task*

Re posture the Army Nurse Corps to deliver patient driven, familycentric evidence based nursing care; provide full spectrum leadership for professional nursing and in support of the Army Medical Department.

#### *Purpose*

Optimize Army Nursing as a key enabler for the Military Health System.

#### *Corps Chief Intent*

I intend to provide continuous, responsive and essential nurse advocacy for the AMEDD's strategic imperatives. All actions and tasks must lead and work toward promoting the wellness of Warriors, their families, and all entrusted to our care; supporting the delivery of patient and family healthcare and ultimately, positioning the Army Nurse Corps as a key enabler for the future of military medicine.

### B. End State

In the near term, the Army Nurse Corps executed effective strategies that provided evidence based nursing care and developed full spectrum leaders: optimized their footprint through aggressive validation of priorities; repostured the force structure to create current and future capacity and capability and maximized performance excellence. Leveraged Strategic Communication that engaged key audiences and created, strengthened, and preserved conditions favorable for the advancement of Army Nurse Corps' interests and objectives. Codified a robust clinical delivery system nested with competencies, capabilities, and evidence based ideology. Transformed Army Nurses into Full Spectrum Leaders, agile and responsive to all conditionsbased missions.

In the far term, the Army Nurse Corps codified and internalized best organizational strategies that provided a relentless focus on organizational improvement, agility and responsiveness.

In the long term, the Army Nurse Corps consistently achieved performance excellence, fostered innovation, built knowledge and capabilities, and insured organizational credibility and sustainability.

## Campaign Plan Objectives

### Leader Development: "Build our bench"

A persistent, sustainable nurse leader succession plan created full spectrum leaders who were adaptive to any conditions based mission; provided a persuasive voice at key echelons of influence in the AMEDD, and innovated doctrine to blueprint the future of the Army Nurse Corps.

### Warrior Care: "Back to basics"

Optimized nursing care delivery systems that wrapped nursing capability around AMEDD strategic goals and mission; Warrior/patient driven/family centric care models embraced evidence based practice to achieve best patient outcomes.

### Evidence-based Management: "Optimize performance"

Evidence based methodology optimized business practices and cost capabilities by blending analysis, measuring, and re designing into daily performance.

### Human Capital: "Portfolio of Expertise"

The Army Nurse Corps footprint is optimized through validation of priorities and the force structure is repostured for conditions based capability and capacity.

## Army Nursing Team Creed

I am a member of the Army Nursing Team[3]

- My patients depend on me and trust me to provide compassionate and proficient care always.
- I nurture the most helpless and vulnerable and offer courage and hope to those in despair.
- I protect the dignity of every individual put in my charge.
- I tend to the physical and psychological wounds of our Warriors and support the health, safety, and welfare of every retired Veteran.
- I am an advocate for family members who support and sustain their Soldier during times of War.
- It is a privilege to care for each of these individuals and I will always strive to be attentive and respectful of their needs and honor their uniquely divine human spirit.

We are the Army Nursing Team

- We honor our professional practice standards and live the Soldier values.
- We believe strength and resiliency in difficult times is the cornerstone of Army Nursing.
- We embrace the diversity of our team and implicitly understand that we must maintain a unified, authentically positive culture and support each other's physical, social, and environmental well being.
- We have a collective responsibility to mentor and foster the professional growth of our newest Team members so they may mentor those who follow.
- We remember those nursing professionals who came before us and honor their legacy, determination, and sacrifice.
- We are fundamentally committed to provide exceptional care to past, present, and future generations who bravely defend and protect our Nation.
- The Army Nursing Team: Courage to Care, Courage to Connect, Courage to Change

---

[3] LTC Leigh McGraw

# Health Care Ethics

Health care ethics (also known as *medical ethics*) is a system of moral principles that apply values and judgments to the practice of medicine. As a scholarly discipline, medical ethics encompasses its practical application in clinical settings as well as work on its history, philosophy, theology, and sociology.

## History

Historically, Western medical ethics may be traced to guidelines on the duty of physicians in antiquity, such as the Hippocratic Oath, and early rabbinic and Christian teachings. In the medieval and early modern period, the field is indebted to Muslim medicine such as Ishaq bin Ali Rahawi (who wrote the Conduct of a Physician, the first book dedicated to medical ethics) and Muhammad ibn Zakariya ar Razi (known as Rhazes in the West), Jewish thinkers such as Maimonides, Roman Catholic scholastic thinkers such as Thomas Aquinas, and the case oriented analysis (casuistry) of Catholic moral theology. These intellectual traditions continue in Catholic, Islamic and Jewish medical ethics.

By the 18th and 19th centuries, medical ethics emerged as a more self conscious discourse. For instance, authors such as Thomas Percival wrote about "medical jurisprudence" and reportedly coined the phrase "medical ethics." Percival's guidelines related to physician consultations have been criticized as being excessively protective of the home physician's reputation. Jeffrey Berlant is one such critic who considers Percival's codes of physician consultations as being an early example of the anti competitive, "guild" like nature of the physician community.[4, 5] In 1847, the American Medical Association adopted its first code of ethics, with this being based in large part upon Percival's work.[6] While the secularized field borrowed largely from Catholic medical ethics, in the 20th century a distinctively liberal Protestant approach was articulated by thinkers such as Joseph Fletcher. In the 1960s and 1970s, building upon liberal theory and procedural justice, much of the discourse of medical ethics went through a dramatic shift and largely reconfigured itself into bioethics.[7]

---

[4] Berlant, Jeffrey (1975). Profession and Monopoly: a study of medicine in the United States and Great Britain. University of California Press. ISBN 0520027345. http://www.pubmedcentral.nih.gov/articlerender.fcgi?artid 1081816.

[5] Percival, Thomas (1849). Medical ethics. John Henry Parker. pp. 49 57 esp section 8 pg.52. http://books.google.com/?id yVUEAAAAQAAJ&printsec frontcover&dq medical+ethics.

[6] Lakhan SE, Hamlat E, McNamee T, Laird C (2009). "Time for a unified approach to medical ethics." Philosophy, Ethics, and Humanities in Medicine 4 (3): 13. doi:10.1186/1747 5341 4 13. PMC 2745426. PMID 19737406. http://www.pubmedcentral.nih.gov/articlerender.fcgi?tool pmcentrez&artid 2745426.

[7] Walter, Klein eds. The Story of Bioethics: From seminal works to contemporary explorations.

Since the 1970s, the growing influence of ethics in contemporary medicine can be seen in the increasing use of Institutional Review Boards to evaluate experiments on human subjects, the establishment of hospital ethics committees, the expansion of the role of clinician ethicists, and the integration of ethics into many medical school curricula.[8]

## Values in Medical Ethics

Six of the values that commonly apply to medical ethics discussions are:

1. **Autonomy** the patient has the right to refuse or choose their treatment. (*Voluntas aegroti suprema lex.*)

2. **Beneficence** a practitioner should act in the best interest of the patient. (*Salus aegroti suprema lex.*)

3. **Non-maleficence** "first, do no harm" (*primum non nocere*).

4. **Justice** concerns the distribution of scarce health resources, and the decision of who gets what treatment (*fairness and equality*).

5. **Dignity** the patient (and the person treating the patient) have the right to dignity.

6. **Truthfulness and honesty** the concept of informed consent has increased in importance since the historical events of the Doctors' Trial of the Nuremberg trials and Tuskegee Syphilis Study.

Values such as these do not give answers as to how to handle a particular situation, but provide a useful framework for understanding conflicts.

When moral values are in conflict, the result may be an ethical dilemma or crisis. Sometimes, no good solution to a dilemma in medical ethics exists, and occasionally, the values of the medical community (i.e., the hospital and its staff) conflict with the values of the individual patient, family, or larger non medical community. Conflicts can also arise between health care providers, or among family members. Some argue for example, that the principles of autonomy and beneficence clash when patients refuse blood transfusions, considering them life saving; and truth telling was not emphasized to a large extent before the HIV era.

---

[8] Lakhan SE, Hamlat E, McNamee T, Laird C (2009). "Time for a unified approach to medical ethics." Philosophy, Ethics, and Humanities in Medicine 4 (3): 13. doi:10.1186/1747 5341 4 13. PMC 2745426. PMID 19737406. http://www.pubmedcentral.nih.gov/articlerender.fcgi?tool pmcentrez&artid 2745426.

# Army Medical Command

The U.S. Army Medical Command (MEDCOM) is a major command of the U.S. Army that provides command and control of the Army's fixed facility medical, dental, and veterinary treatment facilities, providing preventive care, medical research and development and training institutions.

## Structure and Subordinate Commands

MEDCOM is divided into Regional Medical Commands that oversee day to day operations in military treatment facilities, exercising command and control over the medical treatment facilities in their regions. There are currently five of these regional commands:

- Europe Regional Medical Command
- Southern Regional Medical Command
- Northern Regional Medical Command
- Pacific Regional Medical Command
- Western Regional Medical Command.

Additional subordinate commands of MEDCOM include:

- Army Medical Department Center & School (AMEDDC&S)
- U.S. Army Public Health Command (Provisional), (known as the U.S. Army Center for Health Promotion & Preventive Medicine prior to 1 October 2009 {USACHPPM or CHPPM})
- U.S. Army Medical Research and Materiel Command (USAMRMC)
- Warrior Transition Command (WTC)
- U.S. Army Dental Command (DENCOM)

## Operations

### In Garrison (Peacetime)

MEDCOM maintains day to day health care for soldiers, retired soldiers and the families of both. Despite the wide range of responsibilities involved in providing health care in traditional settings as well as on the battlefield, the Army Medical Department's quality of care compares very favorably with that of civilian health organizations, when measured by civilian standards. Many Army medical facilities report on their own quality of care standards on their individual Internet sites.

### Deployments

When Army field hospitals deploy, most clinical professional and support personnel come from MEDCOM's fixed facilities. In addition to support of combat operations, deployments can be for humanitarian assistance, peacekeeping, and other stability and support operations. Under the Professional Officer Filler System (PROFIS), up to 26 percent of MEDCOM physicians and 43 percent of MEDCOM nurses are sent to field units during a full deployment. To replace PROFIS losses, Reserve units and Individual Mobilization Augmentees (non unit reservists) are mobilized to work in medical treatment facilities. The department also provides trained medical specialists to the Army's combat medical units, which are assigned directly to combatant commanders.

Many Army Reserve and Army National Guard units deploy in support of the Army Medical Department. The Army depends heavily on its Reserve component for medical support about 63 percent of the Army's medical forces are in the Reserve component.

## *Army Medical Department*

The Army Medical Department of the U.S. Army (AMEDD) comprises the Army's six medical Special Branches (or "Corps") of officers and medical enlisted soldiers. It was established as the "Army Hospital" in July 1775 to coordinate the medical care required by the Continental Army during the Revolutionary War. The AMEDD is led by the Surgeon General of the U.S. Army, a lieutenant general.

The AMEDD is the U.S. Army's healthcare organization, not a U.S. Army command. The AMEDD is found in all three components of the Army: the Active Army, the U.S. Army Reserve, and the Army National Guard. Its headquarters are at Fort Sam Houston, San Antonio, Texas, which hosts the AMEDD Center and School. Equal numbers of AMEDD senior leaders can be found in Washington D.C., divided between the Pentagon and the Walter Reed Army Medical Center (WRAMC).

The Academy of Health Sciences, under the Army Medical Department Center & School, provides training to the officers and enlisted soldiers of the AMEDD. As a result of BRAC 2005, enlisted medical training was transferred to the new Medical Education and Training Campus, consolidating most military enlisted medical training at Fort Sam Houston.[9]

**Medical Special Branches**

- Medical Corps (MC)
- Nurse Corps (AN)
- Dental Corps (DC)
- Veterinary Corps (VC)
- Medical Service Corps (MS)
- Medical Specialist Corps (AMSC)

## *United States Army Training and Doctrine Command*

Established 1 July 1973, the United States Army Training and Doctrine Command (TRADOC) is an army command of the United States Army headquartered at Fort Monroe, Virginia. It is charged with overseeing training of Army forces, the development of operational doctrine, and the development and procurement of new weapons systems. TRADOC operates 33 schools and centers at 16 Army installations. TRADOC schools conduct 2,734 courses (81 directly in support of mobilization) and 373 language courses. The 2,734 courses include 503,164 seats for 434,424 soldiers; 34,675 other service personnel; 7,824 international soldiers; and 26,241 civilians.[10]

TRADOC MissionThe official mission statement for TRADOC states:

> TRADOC develops the Army's Soldiers and Civilian leaders and designs, develops and integrates capabilities, concepts and doctrine in order to build a campaign capable, expeditionary Army in support of joint warfighting capability through Army Force Generation (ARFORGEN).[11]

---

[9] U.S. Army Medical Department AMEDD Center and School Portal available on the Internet at: http://www.cs.amedd.army.mil/. Additional information specific to the Fort Sam Houston consolidation is available n the Internet at: http://www.aetc.af.mil/shared/media/document/AFD 071026 035.pdf
[10] TRADOC fact sheet available at: http://www.tradoc.army.mil/about.htm
[11] TRADOC commander on ARFORGEN, and the US Army available at: http://www.tradoc.army.mil/about.htm

TRADOC is the official command component that is responsible for training and developing the United States Army.

## TRADOC History

TRADOC was established as a major U.S. Army command on 1 July 1973. The new command, along with the U.S. Army Forces Command (FORSCOM), was created from the Continental Army Command (CONARC) located at Fort Monroe, VA. That action was the major innovation in the Army's post Vietnam reorganization, in the face of realization that CONARC's obligations and span of control were too broad for efficient focus. The new organization functionally realigned the major Army commands in the continental United States. CONARC, and Headquarters, U.S. Army Combat Developments Command (CDC), situated at Fort Belvoir, VA, were discontinued, with TRADOC and FORSCOM at Fort Belvoir assuming the realigned missions. TRADOC assumed the combat developments mission from CDC, took over the individual training mission formerly the responsibility of CONARC, and assumed command from CONARC of the major Army installations in the United States housing Army training center and Army branch schools. FORSCOM assumed CONARC's operational responsibility for the command and readiness of all divisions and corps in the continental U.S. and for the installations where they were based.

Joined under TRADOC, the major Army missions of individual training and combat developments each had its own lineage. The individual training responsibility had belonged, during World War II, to Headquarters Army Ground Forces (AGF). In 1946 numbered Army areas were established in the U.S. under AGF command. At that time, the AGF moved from Washington, D.C. to Fort Monroe, VA. In March 1948, the AGR was replaced at Fort Monroe with the new Office, Chief of Army Field Forces (OCAFF). OCAFF, however, did not command the training establishment. That function was exercised by Headquarters, Department of the Army through the numbered Armies to the corps, division, and Army Training Centers. In February 1955, HQ Continental Army Command (CONARC) replaced OCAFF, assuming its missions as well as the training missions from DA. In January, HQ CONARC was redesignated U.S. Continental Army Command. Combat developments emerged as a formal Army mission in the early 1950s, and OCAFF assumed that role in 1952. In 1955, CONARC assumed the mission. In 1962, HQ U.S. Army Combat Development Command (CDC) was established to bring the combat developments function under one major Army command.[12]

---

[12] TRADOC history available at: http://www.tradoc.army.mil/about.htm

## TRADOC Priorities

1. Leader Development
2. Initial Military Training
3. Concepts and Capabilities Integration
4. Human Capital Enterprise
5. Army Training and Learning Concept
6. Doctrine

# Nursing Fundamentals I

## Subcourse MD0905

This page intentionally left blank.

U.S. ARMY MEDICAL DEPARTMENT CENTER AND SCHOOL
FORT SAM HOUSTON, TEXAS 78234

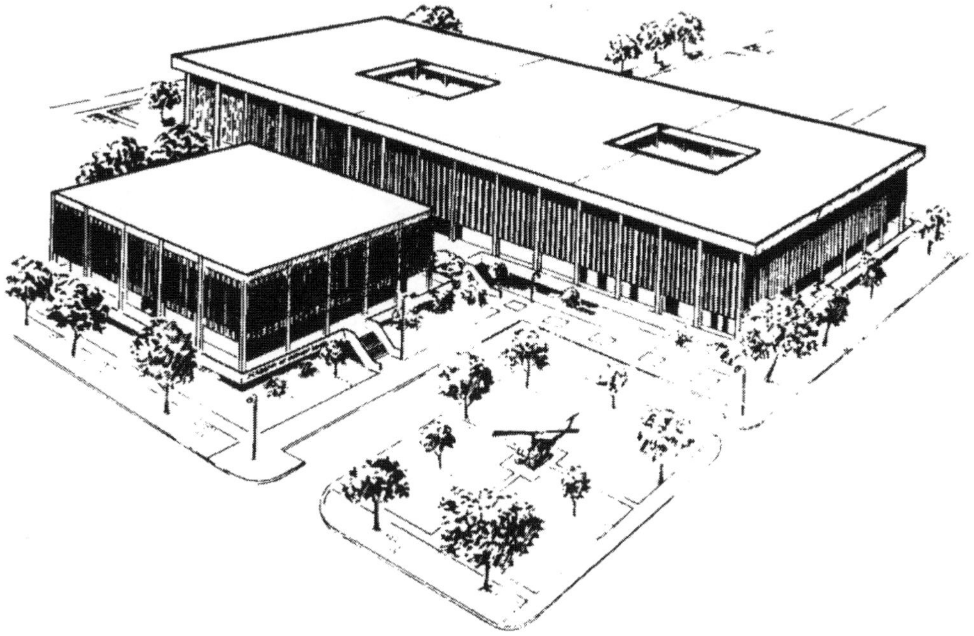

# NURSING FUNDAMENTALS I

SUBCOURSE MD0905 EDITION 100

## DEVELOPMENT

This subcourse is approved for resident and correspondence course instruction. It reflects the current thought of the Academy of Health Sciences and conforms to printed Department of the Army doctrine as closely as currently possible. Development and progress render such doctrine continuously subject to change.

The education specialist responsible for development of this edition was Mr. Joe McNaul, DSN 471-6346 or area code 210-221-6346, Academy of Health Sciences, ATTN: MCCS-HNP, Fort Sam Houston, Texas 78234-6100.

The organization responsible for the subject matter content of this edition is the Nursing Science Division, DSN 471-3086 or area code (210) 221-3086; Director, Phase I, M6 Branch, Academy of Health Sciences, ATTN: MCCS-HNP, Fort Sam Houston, Texas 78234-6100.

## ADMINISTRATION

Students who desire credit hours for this correspondence subcourse must meet eligibility requirements and must enroll through the Nonresident Instruction Branch of the U.S. Army Medical Department Center and School (AMEDDC&S).

Application for enrollment should be made at the Internet website:

http://www.atrrs.army.mil. You can access the course catalog in the upper right corner. Enter School Code 555 for medical correspondence courses. Copy down the course number and title. To apply for enrollment, return to the main ATRRS screen and scroll down the right side for ATRRS Channels. Click on SELF DEVELOPMENT to open the application and then follow the on screen instructions.

For comments or questions regarding enrollment, student records, or shipments, contact the Nonresident Instruction Branch at DSN 471-5877, commercial (210) 221-5877, toll-free 1-800-344-2380; fax: 210-221-4012 or DSN 471-4012, e-mail accp@amedd.army.mil, or write to:

NONRESIDENT INSTRUCTION BRANCH<br>
AMEDDC&S<br>
ATTN: MCCS-HSN<br>
2105 11TH STREET SUITE 4191<br>
FORT SAM HOUSTON TX 78234-5064

## CLARIFICATION OF TERMINOLOGY

When used in this publication, words such as "he," "him," "his," and "men" 'are intended to include both the masculine and feminine genders, unless specifically stated otherwise or when obvious in context.

## TABLE OF CONTENTS

**CORRESPONDENCE COURSE OF THE**
**U.S. ARMY MEDICAL DEPARTMENT CENTER AND SCHOOL**

**SUBCOURSE MED905**

# NURSING FUNDAMENTALS I

## INTRODUCTION

Never before has there been a greater need for nurses. Never before has health care delivery challenged the nurse's commitment, knowledge, or technical competence more. Issues influencing current health-care delivery focus on promoting wellness, preventing illness, and rehabilitation to increase the patient's independence.
This subcourse will present theory and concepts the person beginning the study of nursing will need to know in order to develop the knowledge and competence demanded by the complexity of the changing health care system.

Subcourse Components:

This subcourse consists of 6 lessons:

Lesson 1. Patient Relations.

Lesson 2. The Adult Patient Care Unit.

Lesson 3. Advanced Principles of Patient Hygiene.

Lesson 4. Body Mechanics.

Lesson 5. Active and Passive Range of Motion Exercises.

Lesson 6. Environmental Health and The Practical Nurse.

Credit Awarded:

Upon successful completion of this subcourse, you will be awarded 12 credit hours.

Procedures for Subcourse Completion:

You are encouraged to complete the subcourse lesson by lesson. When you have completed all of the lessons to your satisfaction, fill out the examination answer sheet and mail it to the AMEDDC&S along with the Student Comment Sheet in the envelope provided. Be sure that your name, rank, social security number, and return address are on all correspondence sent to the AMEDDC&S. You will be notified by return mail of the examination results. Your grade on the exam will be your rating for the subcourse.

Study Suggestions:

Here are some suggestions that may be helpful to you in completing this subcourse:

--Read and study each lesson carefully.

--Complete the subcourse lesson by lesson. After completing each lesson, work the exercises at the end of the lesson, marking your answers in this booklet.

--After completing each set of lesson exercises, compare your answers with those on the solution sheet, which follows the exercises. If you have answered an exercise incorrectly, check the reference cited after the answer on the solution sheet to determine why your response was not the correct one.

--As you successfully complete each lesson, go on to the next. When you. have completed all of the lessons, complete the examination. Mark your answers in the examination booklet; then transfer your responses to the examination answer sheet using a #2 pencil.

Student Comment Sheet:

Be sure to provide us with your suggestions and criticisms by filling out the Student Comment Sheet (found at the back of this booklet) and returning it to us with your examination answer sheet. Please review this comment sheet before studying this subcourse. In this way, you will help us to improve the quality of this subcourse.

## UNIVERSAL BODY SUBSTANCE PRECAUTIONS

### Prevention of Transmission of Human Immunodeficiency Virus and Other Blood-Borne Pathogens in Health Care Settings

Only blood, semen, vaginal secretions, and possibly breast milk have been implicated in transmission of human immunodeficiency virus (HIV), hepatitis B virus (HBV), and other blood-borne pathogens.

Blood is the single most important source of transmission of blood-borne pathogens in health care settings. Infection control efforts must focus on preventing exposures to blood.

Although the risk is unknown, universal precautions also apply to tissues and to cerebrospinal fluid, synovial fluid, pleural fluid, peritoneal fluid, and amniotic fluid.

Universal precautions do not apply to feces, nasal secretions, sputum, sweat, tears, urine, and vomitus unless they contain visible blood. Although universal precautions do not apply to these body substances, the wise nurse wears gloves for protection from other infections.

Precautions are used for *all* patients. (*Reason:* It is impossible to know which patients are infected with such conditions as HIV, HBV, or other infectious agents.)

Gloves are worn *whenever* the health care worker may come in contact with blood, body fluids containing blood, and other body fluids to which universal precautions apply. (*Reason:* Diseases can be carried in the body substances.)

Wear gloves *at all times* if you have any break in the skin of your hands. If you have an exudative condition, such as weeping dermatitis, you must be evaluated before working with patients and patient care equipment. (*Reason:* You may be at great risk of contracting a disease; you might also spread disease.)

Change gloves after each contact with a client. (*Reason:* The gloves may be contaminated.)

Wash your hands and skin surfaces immediately and thoroughly if they are contaminated with blood or body fluids. (*Reason:* Proper washing will help to stop the spread of infection.)

Wear a gown or apron when clothing could become soiled. (*Reason:* To prevent spread of infection to yourself or others.)

Wear a mask and eye protection if splashing is possible. Hospital protocol will determine what type of eye protection is required for each specific case. (*Reason:* Infection could enter your body through the mucous membranes of your mouth or nose or through your eyes.)

Dispose of sharp objects carefully. Do not recap or break needles. Needles and sharp objects are placed in a special container after use. (*Reason:* There is a possibility of accidental finger stick. It is important to protect yourself and housekeeping personnel.)

If you have an on-the-job accident that causes a break in the skin, notify your nursing supervisor *immediately*. (*Reason:* Immediate precautions must be taken to protect you.)

Special care is taken of a deceased patient's body. (*Reason:* To prevent leakage of body substances. It is safer to assume that all patients are infectious.)

All health care workers who perform or assist in vaginal or cesarean delivery should wear gloves and gowns when handling the placenta or the infant until blood and amniotic fluid have been removed from the infant's skin. Gloves should be worn until after postdelivery care of the umbilical cord.

Pregnant health care workers are not known to be at greater risk of contracting HIV infection than health care workers who are not pregnant; however, if a health care worker develops HIV infection during pregnancy, the infant is at risk. Because of this risk, pregnant health care workers should be especially familiar with and strictly adhere to precautions to minimize the risk of HIV transmission.

*(Adapted from Centers for Disease Control: Recommendations for prevention of HIV transmission in health care settings. MMWR 36: Suppl. 25: 1987. Centers for Disease Control: Update: Universal precautions for prevention or transmission of human immunodeficiency virus, hepatitis B virus, and other blood-borne pathogens in health-care settings. MMWR 37: 24, 1988)*

***END OF UNIVERSAL BODY SUBSTANCES***

## LESSON ASSIGNMENT

**LESSON 1** Patient Relations

**TEXT ASSIGNMENT** Paragraphs 1-1 through 1-31

**LESSON OBJECTIVES** After completing this lesson, you should be able to:

1-1. Identify basic concepts of health.

1-2. Identify basic human needs.

1-3. Identify examples of Maslow's Hierarchy of Needs.

1-4. Identify purposes of human communication.

1-5. Identify components of the human communication system.

1-6. Identify methods of verbal and nonverbal communication.

1-7. Recognize appropriate techniques of communication with patients.

1-8. Recognize appropriate techniques of interviewing patients.

1-9. Define and identify critical elements of therapeutic communication.

1-10. Identify nursing interventions needed to communicate with the patient who is blind, deaf, or speaks a foreign language.

1-11. Identify factors influencing whether a person seeks or avoids professional help.

1-12. Identify factors causing stress in a hospital.

1-13. Identify the stages of illness.

1-14 Recognize common emotional reactions to illness and hospitalization

1-15. Define and identify factors of transcultural nursing.

1-16. Identify sociocultural beliefs about illness, to include causes, cures, and nursing implications.

1-17. Match religious denominations with appropriate beliefs and nursing implications.

**SUGGESTION**

After studying the assignment, complete the exercises at the end of the lesson. These exercises will help you to achieve the lesson objectives.

# LESSON 1

# PATIENT RELATIONS

## Section I. BASIC HUMAN NEEDS AND PRINCIPLES OF HEALTH

### 1-1. INTRODUCTION

Health is one of our most precious possessions. The preservation of health is met through the satisfaction of our basic human needs. Understanding the basic needs of people, therefore, is essential for the practical nurse in planning for and meeting the needs of the patient.

### 1-2. PRINCIPLES OF HEALTH

a. **Definition of Health**.

(1) An individual's concept of health is a very personal thing. One person may consider himself to be healthy whenever he is not physically ill, while another may consider himself to be healthy only when he is emotionally and physically "at his best." A person's notion of health is influenced by a number of different factors or experiences, such as family background, self-concept, religion, past experiences, and socioeconomic status. It is important that you, as a practical nurse, keep this in mind when dealing with your patient's, as well as your own, feelings and interactions.

(2) For purposes of this subcourse, we will define health as a state of complete physical, mental, and social well-being, not merely the absence of disease or infirmity.

b. **Total Health**. Although the absence of disease and illness is, by anyone's definition, essential to good health, it is, by no means, the only factor. Total health includes all of the following aspects as well:

(1) Social health. A sense of responsibility for the health and welfare of others.

(2) Mental health. A mind that grows, reasons, and adjusts to life situations.

(3) Emotional health. Feelings and actions that bring one satisfaction.

(4) Spiritual health. Inner peace and security in one's spiritual faith.

## 1-3. THE HEALTH-ILLNESS CONTINUUM

a. The individual's state of health is one of continual change. He moves back and forth from health to illness and back to health again. His condition is rarely constant. He may wake up feeling great, develop a headache mid-morning, and feel fine again by noon. The health-illness continuum (see figure 1-1) illustrates this process of change, in which the individual experiences various states of health and illness (ranging from extremely good health to death) that fluctuate throughout his life.

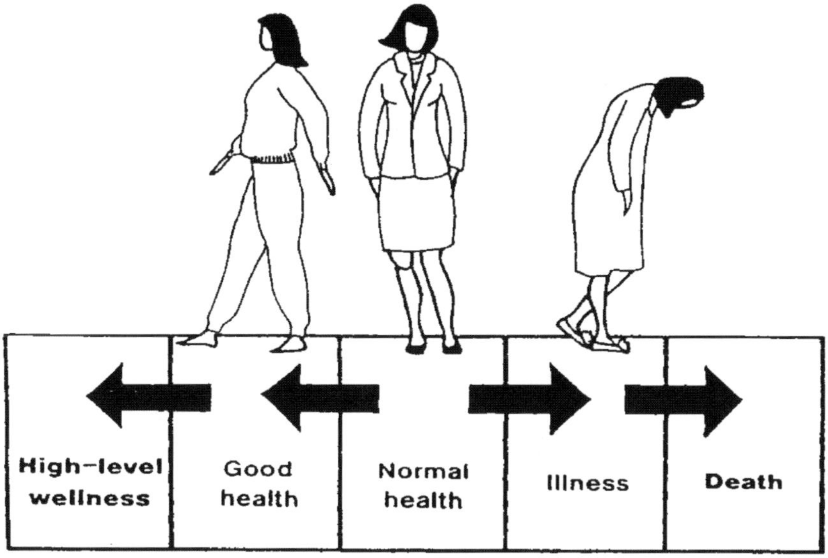


Figure 1-1. The health-illness continuum.

b. As we previously stated, health, just as life itself, is a process of continual change. And we must continually adapt to these changes in our lives in order to maintain good health and well-being. It is our adaptation or response to that change, rather than the change itself, that affects our health. For example, two students just found out about a big test tomorrow, for which they are completely unprepared. One student responds to this stressful situation (stressor) by going home, getting his books out, and starting to study. The other student breaks out into a sweat, and spends most of the evening fretting over this outrage and imagining what will happen to him if he doesn't pass the test. No doubt, this student is doing more damage to his health than is his friend. And, considering the time and energy he is expending on worrying (and not studying), he may experience even more stress when they receive their grades!

c. Adaptation and effective functioning, even in the presence of chronic disease, can be considered a state of wellness. A person may be in perfect physical condition, but feel too tired and "blue" to go to work, while his co-worker, a diabetic, is at work, functioning fully and accomplishing his job. Which of these two people is at a higher level on the health-illness continuum?

**NOTE**: Death occurs when adaptation fails completely, and there is irreversible damage to the body.

## 1-4. ADAPTING TO CHANGE

The individual's state of health is determined by the ability to adapt to changes in the following dimensions:

a. Developmental--changes in a person's behavior and ability, which are associated with increasing age.

b. Psychosocial--the development of the personality, social attitudes, and skills.

c. Cultural--changes in or development of beliefs and values held by the individual's family or culture.

d. Physiological--changes in body function.

## 1-5. POSITIVE HEALTH HABITS

Regardless of one's definition of health, the individual who practices the following positive health habits on a regular basis is certainly at an advantage.

a. A balanced diet with adequate caloric intake.

b. Efficient elimination.

c. Regular exercise.

d. Adequate sleep, rest periods, and relaxation periods.

e. Regular medical checkups.

f. Regular dental checkups.

g. Maintenance of good posture.

h. Good grooming habits.

## 1-6. CATEGORIES OF BASIC HUMAN NEEDS

a. **Physical Needs**. These are closely related to body functions and are sometimes referred to as primary or physiological drives. Physical needs include:

(1) Food.

(2) Water.

(3) Oxygen.

(4) Elimination.

(5) Clothing and shelter for body warmth and protection.

(6) Activity, or sensory and motor stimulation, including sex, physical exercise, and rest.

b. **Emotional Needs**. Emotional needs are closely interwoven with physical needs and are met in interaction with significant others. They include:

(1) Love, including approval and esteem.

(2) Importance, including recognition and respect.

**NOTE**: This applies to the patient's perception of the nurse's feelings toward him. For example, if your patient feels that you do not approve of or respect him, he may become very demanding, or he may withdraw and not cooperate with your efforts to make him healthy again.

(3) Adequacy, including self-sufficiency and the need to be needed and wanted.

(4) Productivity, including work and creative pursuits.

c. **Social Needs**.

Social needs grow out of the culture and society of which one is a member. They include:

(1) Identification or belonging.

(2) Education or learning.

(3) Recreation or play.

(4) Religion or worship.

**NOTE**: Remember that all human behavior is aimed toward the satisfaction of basic human needs.

## 1-7. MASLOW'S HIERARCHY OF NEEDS

Psychologist Abraham Maslow defined basic human needs as a hierarchy, a progression from simple physical needs to more complex emotional needs (see figure 1-2).

a. **Types of Needs**.

(1) Physiological--food, shelter, water, sleep, oxygen.

(2) Safety--security, stability, order, physical safety.

(3) Love and belonging--affection, identification, companionship.

(4) Esteem and recognition--self-esteem, self-respect, prestige, success, esteem of others.

(5) Self-actualization--self-fulfillment, achieving one's own capabilities.

(6) Aesthetic--beauty, harmony, spiritual.

b. **Relationship Between Levels of Needs.**

(1) According to Maslow, the basic physiological needs related to survival (food, water, etc.) must be met first of all.

(2) These basic physiological needs have a greater priority over those higher on the pyramid. They must be met before the person can move on to higher level needs. In other words, a person who is starving will not be concentrating on building his self-esteem. A patient in severe pain will not be concerned with improving his interpersonal relationships.

(3) Generally speaking, each lower level must be achieved before the next higher level(s) can be focused upon.

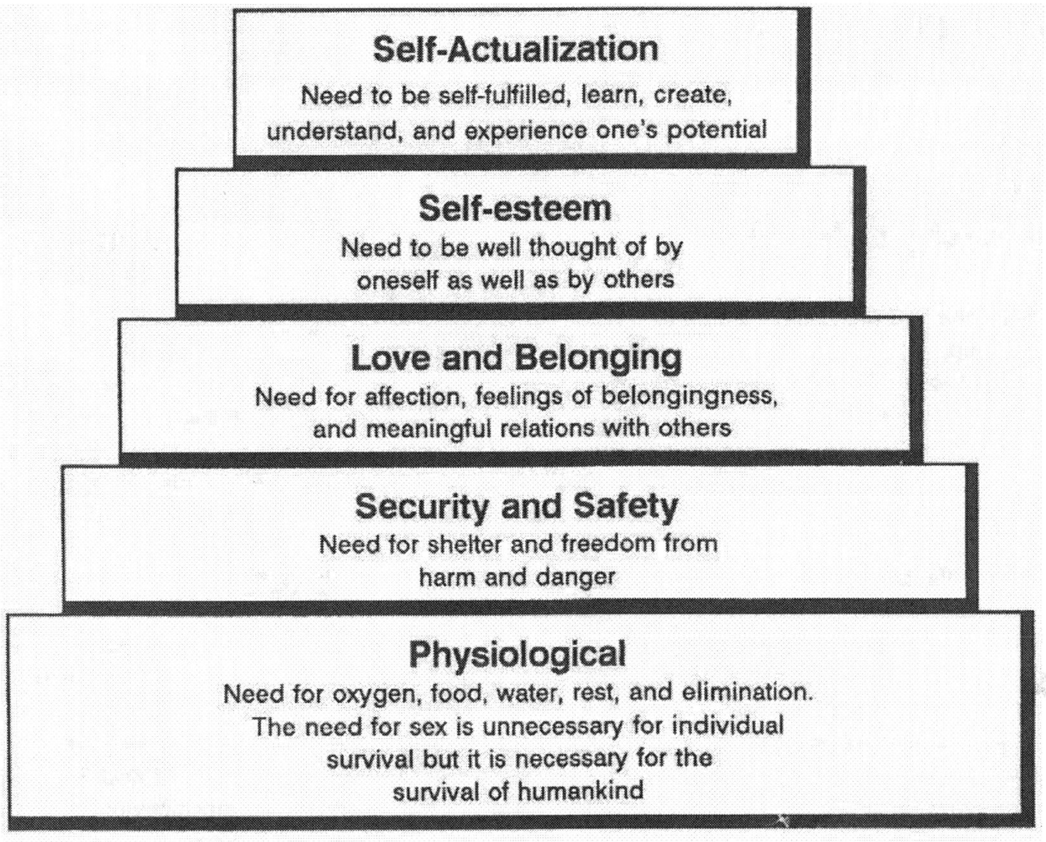


Figure 1-2. Maslow's hierarchy of needs.

c. **Relationship Between Levels of Needs.**

(1) According to Maslow, the basic physiological needs related to survival (food, water, and so forth.) must be met first of all.

(2) These basic physiological needs have a greater priority over those higher on the pyramid. They must be met before the person can move on to higher level needs. In other words, a person who is starving will not be concentrating on building his self-esteem. A patient in severe pain will not be concerned with improving his interpersonal relationships.

(3) Generally speaking, each lower level must be achieved before the next higher level(s) can be focused upon.

## 1-8. COMPARISON OF BASIC HUMAN NEEDS AND MASLOW'S HIERARCHY OF NEEDS

The categories of Maslow's hierarchy are closely related to the basic human needs discussed in paragraph 1-6. Table 1-1 contains a comparison.

| **Maslow's Hierarchy of Needs** | **Basic Human Needs** |
|---|---|
| Physiological: Food, shelter, water, sleep, oxygen<br><br>Safety: Security, stability, order, physical Safety | Physical Needs: Food, water, oxygen, Elimination, clothing and shelter for body warmth and protection, activity, or sensory and motor stimulation, including sex, physical exercise, and rest |
| Love and Belonging: Affection, identification, companionship<br><br>Esteem and Recognition: Self-esteem, self-respect, prestige, success, esteem of others | Emotional Needs: Love, including approval and esteem, importance, including recognition and respect, adequacy, including self-sufficiency and the need to be needed and wanted, productivity, including work an creative pursuits |
| Self-actualization: Self-fulfillment, achieving one's capabilities<br><br>Aesthetic: Beauty, harmony, spiritual | Social Needs: Identification or belonging, education or learning, religion or spiritual, recreation or play |

Table 1-1. Comparison of basic human needs and Maslow's hierarchy of needs.

a. Physical needs are roughly equivalent to Maslow's physiological and safety needs.

b. Emotional needs are roughly equivalent to Maslow's love and belonging and esteem and recognition needs.

c. Social needs are roughly equivalent to Maslow's self-actualization and aesthetic needs.

## 1-9. CLOSING

Remember that human needs are not constant; they are fluid and changing with first one, then another, taking priority. What may start as a basic need for food can take on social and personal significance. Your care plan as well as your patience are aimed toward the satisfaction of the patient's needs. He has common needs because he is a person; he has individual needs because he is unique; he has special needs because he is sick. The Practical Nurse supplies the help that is required to meet the patient's needs during the stressful periods of hospitalization and recuperation.

## Section II. COMMUNICATION SKILLS

### 1-10. INTRODUCTION

If you were to try to explain the process of human interaction, you might define it as a huge and very complex communication system. Nevertheless, it is essential that you develop and maintain an understanding of the methods and skills of communication in order to meet the needs of the patient. The quality of care you can provide is, in many ways, dependent on the quality of communication that exists between you and your patient. Through your direct contact, the patient must perceive your intentions of support and your positive expectations. You must accurately assess the patient's physical and emotional symptoms. Communication has only taken place if the message being sent was accurately received.

### 1-11. PURPOSES OF COMMUNICATION

a. **Major Purpose**. To send, receive, interpret, and respond appropriately and clearly to a message, an interchange of information.

b. **Supportive Purposes**.

(1) To correct the information a person has about himself and others.

(2) To provide the satisfaction or pleasure of expressing oneself.

### 1-12. ESSENTIAL COMPONENTS OF THE HUMAN COMMUNICATION SYSTEM

The essential components of communication are:

a. Sender--the originator or source of the idea.

b. Message--the idea.

c. Channel--the means of transmitting (either verbally or nonverbally) the idea.

d. Receiver--someone to receive and interpret the message.

e. Feedback--the response to the message.

## 1-13. VERBAL AND NONVERBAL METHODS OF COMMUNICATION

a. **Verbal Communication**. Verbal communication refers to the use of the spoken word to acknowledge, amplify, confirm, contrast, or contradict other verbal and nonverbal messages.

b. **Nonverbal Communication**. Nonverbal communication refers to an exchange of information without the exchange of spoken words (facial expressions, body language, etc.).

c. **Essential Relationship**. Verbal communication is always accompanied by nonverbal expression. Even no expression tells the other person something.

## 1-14. METHODS OF NONVERBAL COMMUNICATION

a. **Rapport**. The harmonious feeling experienced by two people who hold one another in mutual respect, acceptance, and understanding.

b. **Empathy**.

(1) Empathy is that degree of understanding, which allows one person to experience how, another feels in a particular situation.

(2) Empathy is neither sympathy (feeling sorry for another person) nor compassion (that quality of love or tenderness that causes one person to suffer along with another).

c. **Body Language.** Remember that actions speak louder than words. A person will generally pay more attention to what you do than what you say. Think about the following nonverbal messages and what they might reveal.

(1) Facial expressions (smile, frown, blank look, grimace).

(2) Gestures/mannerisms (fidgeting, toe tapping, clenched fists).

(3) Eye behaviors (avoiding eye contact, staring, wide eyes).

(4) Use (and avoidance) of touch or physical contact.

(5) Posture (erect, slouching, leaning toward/away from someone).

(6) Walk.

d. **Silence.** Silence can be an extremely effective communication tool. It can be used to express a wide range of feelings.

(1) Silence can be used to communicate the deepest kind of love and devotion, when words are not needed.

(2) Silence can be a cold and rejecting sort of punishment, the "silent treatment" received for coming home late or forgetting an anniversary.

(3) Silence can be used in an interview or conversation to encourage the other person to "open up." Conversely, it can be used to intentionally create anxiety and discomfort in the other person.

e. **Listening**. As a patient speaks, think about what he must be feeling. Sometimes, as a listener, you must cut through layers of words to get to the real message. You must read between the lines. Pick up the underlying meaning of the message (intent); don't rely entirely upon the obvious or superficial meaning (content).

## 1-15. GUIDELINES FOR COMMUNICATING WITH PATIENTS AND THEIRFAMILIES

a. Convey to the patient and family that they are important to you and that you want to help them. There are many ways to do this; you must do what is comfortable and natural for you. However, there are some things everyone can do.

b. Convey honesty and trustworthiness.

(1) Try not to overwhelm the patient with embarrassing or personal questions. When it is necessary to ask personal questions, explain why and keep it short and matter-of-fact.

(2) Don't make promises you can't keep. If you say you are going to do something, make every effort to do it or see that it gets done.

(3) Try to be there when you say you will. If you are late, explain why.

c. Communicate with each patient as an individual. (This is especially important in a hospital setting, where patients often experience a loss of identity.) In order to do so, you must try to get to know the patient. Listen to him. Put yourself in his place.

d. Accept and respect the patient despite the symptoms of his illness.

## 1-16. TECHNIQUES FOR COMMUNICATING WITH PATIENTS

a. **Establishing the Setting.**

(1) Provide a comfortable environment (lighting, temperature, furnishings).

(2) Establish a relaxed, unhurried setting.

(3) Sit down when speaking to the patient. Although you probably have dozens of things you need to be doing at that moment, try to relax. Don't stand at the doorway or sit on the edge of your seat, as if you are preparing to jump and run as soon as you can get away.

(4) Face the speaker and maintain eye contact.

(5) Provide for privacy.

(6) Avoid interruptions and other distracting influences.

b. **Verbal Communication Skills**.

(1) Let the patient do the talking.

(2) Keep questions brief and simple.

(3) Use language that is understandable to the patient. Avoid acronyms and medical/nursing jargon if the patient is nonmedical.

(4) Ask one question at a time. Give the patient time to answer.

(5) Clarify patient responses to questions, not just for your <u>own</u> use, but also to let the patient know that you are listening (be sure you really <u>are)</u> and that you understand.

(6) Avoid leading questions. You want the patient to tell you what he is feeling, not what he thinks you want to hear. So avoid putting words in his mouth. For example, it might be better to ask, "How are you feeling?" rather than "I suppose you're feeling rested after your nap."

(7) Avoid how or why questions; they tend to be intimidating.

(8) Avoid the use of cliché statements like, "Don't worry; it'll be all right." or "Your doctor knows best."

(9) Avoid questions, which require only a simple "yes" or "no" response. You want to encourage the patient to talk to you.

(10) Avoid interrupting the patient. If you need to ask a question, wait until he has completed his thought.

c. **Interviewing Techniques**. The following terms represent skills often used to foster better communication. Before using these techniques, remember that you must do what feels comfortable and natural to you. Even though you may have the best of intentions, if you do not sound sincere, what are the chances of someone really opening up to you? Also, keep in mind that your patients are individuals; if you sense that a particular patient may not respond well to a certain technique, you are probably right.

(1) Reflection. Repeating content or feelings. You might simply repeat what the patient has said, to give him time to mull it over or to encourage him to respond. Or, and often more effectively, you can reflect on what you think the patient is feeling. "It sounds like you're concerned about your family." or "I don't think you're very happy about this." By reflecting on his feelings, you may be encouraging him to talk about something he may have been hesitant to bring up himself. Or you may be helping the patient to identify his own feelings about something.

(2) Restating. Rephrasing a question or summarizing a statement. "You're asking why these tests are needed?" or "In other words, you think you're being treated like a child."

(3) Facilitation. Occasional brief responses, which encourage the speaker to continue. A nod of the head; an occasional verbal cue, such as "go on" or "I see;" and maintaining eye contact throughout the conversation all imply that you are listening and that you understand.

(4) Open-ended questions. Questions that encourage the patient to expound on a topic. If you want to encourage the patient to speak freely, you might ask "How are you feeling?" rather than "Are you in pain?"

(5) Closed-ended questions. Questions, which focus the patient on a specific topic. If you want a short, straight answer, ask a question which will allow only for a direct response, such as "When was your accident?" or "Do you have pain after eating?"

(6) Silence. A quiet period that allows a patient to gather his thoughts. Of course, this would be an occasional practice, used when you feel that the patient could use a little time to think about his response to a question or just to think.

(7) Broad openings. A few words to encourage the patient to further discuss a topic; for example, "and after that..." or "you were saying..."

(8) Clarification. Statements or questions that verify a patient's concern or point. "I'm a bit confused about...Do you think you could go over that again please?"

## 1-17. THERAPEUTIC COMMUNICATION

a. Practicing therapeutic communication is in many ways simply developing a good bedside manner. When your patient asks you a question or discusses something with you, be careful to respond in a helpful and caring manner. By encouraging the patient to speak up, you are probably helping him/her to decrease his level of stress and thereby his recovery time. Study the techniques discussed in paragraphs 1-15 and 1-16. Become familiar enough with them so that they become a natural part of your conversations.

b. When your patient communicates with you, you must be able to correctly observe, evaluate, and respond. Your knowledge, understanding, and skill in human relations will enable you to do so.

## 1-18. CRITICAL ELEMENTS OF EFFECTIVE THERAPEUTIC COMMUNICATION

a. Be able to decipher the patient's message. Get to know the patient well enough to discover the underlying meaning (intent) of his/her communication. Be alert and perceptive enough to pick up the correct message. Many people feel uncomfortable talking about their feelings, especially if they are trying to be "good patients." Learn to "read between the lines."

b. Be realistic in your relationships with people; avoid making assumptions or judgments about your patients' behavior. If you have negative thoughts about something a patient says or does, try to keep in mind that he is an adult, responsible for making his own decisions. You do not want him to feel he must conceal anything from you. You want him to see that you will accept him for what he is; you will allow him his own identity.

c. Be emotionally mature enough to postpone the satisfaction of your own needs in deference to the patient's. Find sources other than the therapeutic relationship to meet your own needs.

## 1-19. NURSING INTERVENTION WITH PATIENTS WITH SPECIAL COMMUNICATION NEEDS

a. **Blind Patients**.

(1) Always speak to the patient when you enter the room so he will know who is there.

(2) Speak directly to the patient; do not turn your back.

(3) Speak to the patient in a normal tone of voice; he is blind, not deaf.

(4) Speak to the patient before touching him/her.

(5) Offer to help with arrangements for patients who may enjoy hearing tapes or reading Braille literature.

b. **Deaf Patients**.

(1) Look directly at the patient when speaking with him/her.

(2) Do not cover your mouth when speaking because the patient may read lips.

(3) If the patient does not lip-read, charts with pictures may be used, or simply writing your questions or comments on a piece of paper may be helpful.

(4) Charts with hand signs are available at the local society for deafness and/or hearing preservation.

c. **Patients Speaking a Foreign Language**.

(1) Obtain a translator if possible. The Red Cross or the Patient Administration Division (PAD) may be of assistance.

(2) Have a chart with basic phrases in English and the foreign language.

(3) Consider using charts with pictures.

## 1-20. CLOSING

When communicating with patients, each Practical Nurse has to find the ways that are the most effective for the people and circumstances concerned. If the Practical Nurse tries to express care and concern for the patient and can communicate well verbally and nonverbally, the nurse-patient relationship will thrive.

# Section III. REACTION TO STRESS AND HOSPITALIZATION

## 1-21. INTRODUCTION

The patient who is entering a hospital is under many emotional pressures. Fear of death, disfigurement, pain, or a prolonged illness, and loss of control of the surrounding environment are just a few of the emotional concerns being faced. People react to stress in many ways. The Practical Nurse must be able to recognize the signs and symptoms of stress and identify the coping mechanisms being utilized by the patient in order to provide effective nursing care.

## 1-22. FACTORS INFLUENCING WHETHER A PERSON WILL SEEK OR AVOID PROFESSIONAL HELP

Some of the factors that influence a person seeking or avoiding professional help are:

a. The degree and extent of symptom distress.

b. Expectation of return to health if treatment is instituted.

c. Fear of diagnostic and treatment procedures.

d. Fear of discovery of serious illness.

e. The self-concept that one is always healthy.

## 1-23. FACTORS CAUSING STRESS IN THE HOSPITAL

Some of the factors that cause stress in the hospital are:

a. **Unfamiliarity of surroundings**.

(1) Having strangers sleep in the same room.

(2) Having to eat cold or tasteless food.

(3) Being awakened in the night by the nurse.

b. **Loss of independence**.

(1) Having to eat at different times than usual.

(2) Having to wear a hospital gown.

(3) Not having the call light answered.

c. **Separation from spouse**.

d. **Separation from family**.

e. **Financial problems**.

f. **Isolation from other people**.

(1) Having an unfriendly roommate.

(2) Not having friends visit.

(3) Having staff in too much of a hurry to talk, or more importantly, listen.

g. **Lack of information**.

(1) Not having questions answered by staff members.

(2) Having nurses or doctors who talk too fast. Nervousness and preoccupation often make it difficult to fully concentrate on what is being said. Needless to say, patients often have plenty on their minds, so it is crucial that you explain things patiently and slowly and be prepared to repeat instructions and explanations. Do not assume that because you have explained something once, your job is done.

(3) Not knowing the reasons for (or the results of) treatments.

h. **Threat of severe illness**.

(1) Fear that appearance will be changed after hospitalization.

(2) Being hospitalized after an accident and suspecting the worst.

(3) Thinking he/she may have cancer.

i. **Problems with medications**.

(1) Having medications cause discomfort (that is., chemotherapy).

(2) Not getting relief from pain.

(3) Not getting pain medication when needed.

## 1-24. STAGES OF THE ILLNESS EXPERIENCE

a. **Denial or Disbelief in Being Ill.**

(1) Patient may avoid, refuse, or even forget needed care.

(2) Patient may appear to flee toward health in trying to escape illness.

b. **Acceptance of Being Ill.**

(1) Becomes dependent on health care personnel.

(2) Focuses attention on symptoms and the illness.

(3) Gradually becomes less dependent.

c. **Recovery, Rehabilitation, or Convalescence**.

(1) May be a short or long period, depending on how much the patient's life-style must change as a result of the illness.

(2) Patient goes through a process of resolving his/her perceived loss or impairment of function.

## 1-25. EMOTIONAL RESPONSES TO ILLNESS AND HOSPITALIZATION

a. **Fear.**

(1) An emotional response characterized by an expectation of harm or unpleasantness.

(2) Usually associated with behavior that attempts to avoid or flee a threatening situation.

(3) Patient is usually aware of the specific danger and has some understanding into the reasons for the fear.

(4) Common indications of fear include:

(a) Tachycardia (rapid heart rate).

(b) Dry mouth.

(c) Constipation.

(d) Hypertension.

(e) Increased perspiration.

(f) The "fight or flight" reaction (alertness and readiness for action in order to avoid or escape harm).

b. **Anxiety**.

(1) An emotional response characterized by feelings of uneasiness and apprehension of a probable danger or misfortune.

(2) Patient who is anxious usually is unaware of the cause of the anxiety.

(3) Behaviors are similar to those seen with the fear, but are not usually as dramatic.

(4) Because the patient does not know its specific cause, he/she usually focuses on the physiologic symptoms of anxiety, to include:

(a) Fatigue.

(b) Insomnia.

(c) Diarrhea or constipation.

(d) Urgency.

(e) Nausea.

(f) Anorexia.

(g) Excessive perspiration.

c. **Stress**.

(1) A state of strain or tension.

(2) Occurs in situations, which require an increased and often prolonged effort to adjust.

(3) Any factor that disturbs the physical, psychological, or physiological homeostasis of the body may be stressful.

(4) As with fear, the body tries to rid itself of the factor causing the stress.

(5) Physical signs of stress include:

(a) Ulcers.

(b) Hair loss.

(c) Insomnia.

d. **Over Dependency or Feelings of Helplessness.**

(1) Over dependency is a response characterized by feelings of helplessness while trying to search for help and understanding (to an extent beyond what is considered normal).

(2) Helplessness is a response characterized by feelings of being unable to avoid an unpleasant experience.

(3) While healthy people may show some degree of dependence on others during illness, this dependence often increases to the point of being harmful to the patient.

(4) The over dependent patient may be fearful or angry.

## 1-26. CLOSING

There are as many reactions to illness as there are patients. Your kindness and understanding will help your patient to go through the hospitalization experience with a minimum of stress and anxiety.

# Section IV. TRANSCULTURAL FACTORS INFLUENCING NURSING CARE

## 1-27. INTRODUCTION

Transcultural nursing refers to the nursing care of all patients, taking into consideration their religious and sociocultural backgrounds. There are many variables to consider in giving nursing care to a person of a race, religion, or culture different from your own. Respect for the patient, however, is something all aspects of transcultural nursing have in common.

## 1-28. MAJOR FACTORS IN TRANSCULTURAL NURSING

a. Nutrition and dietary practices.

b. Beliefs about illness, its causes and cures.

c. Disorders specific to a particular group, such as the high incidence of sickle cell anemia among the Blacks.

d. Specific anatomical characteristics (e.g, stature, skin tone, hair texture).

e. Religious beliefs about illness and death.

## 1-29. VARIABLES RELATING TO THE TRANSCULTURAL ASPECTS OF NURSING

Some of the factors are:

a. Cultural background of the nurse; differences and similarities between the patient and the nurse.

b. Definition of health and illness accepted by a specific culture; concepts relating to the causes of illness and injury.

c. Folk medicine practices.

d. Attitudes toward health care, relationships, and interactions (e.g., personal space, eye contact).

e. Economic level of the patient and family (socioeconomic status).

f. Environmental factors and related disorders (e.g., ghetto living, lead poisoning).

g. Specific names and terms related to the illness or disorder (e.g.,"bad blood," "mal ojo"); use of slang.

h. Language differences between the health care staff and the patient and family.

i. Modesty and concept of the human body.

j. Reactions to pain, aging, and death.

k. Attitudes about childbirth, abortion, sexual expression, children born to unmarried parents, and homosexuality.

l. Attitudes about mental illness and retardation.

m. Diets in relation to religious and cultural practices; dietary taboos.

n. Attitudes about physical appearance and obesity; adaptation to special therapeutic diets.

o. Importance of religion and religious practices.

p. Religious practices in illness and death; specific prohibitions.

q. Group identity; importance and type of family structure; cohesiveness within the group; traditional roles of men and women.

r. "Visibility" of ethnic background (that is, Black, Oriental).

s. Disorders specific to a cultural group (that is, Tay-Sachs, sickle cell anemia).

t. Attitudes about school; educational level and aspirations of most members of the group.

u. Predominant occupations within the group; role models.

v. "Americanization" of younger members.

w. Numbers of people belonging to that group in the same geographic area as the health care facility.

x. Prejudices within a cultural group relating to other members of the same group.

y. Stereotypes about other cultural/ethnic groups.

z. Mixed families (mixed races, religions, or cultural backgrounds).

**1-30. SOCIOCULTURAL BELIEFS ABOUT ILLNESS, ITS CAUSES, AND CURES**

a. **Examples of Differences in Beliefs About the Causes of Illness**.

(1) <u>Japanese Shintoist</u>.

(a) Man is inherently good.

(b) Illness is caused when the person comes into contact with pollutants, such as blood or a corpse.

(2) <u>Native Americans</u>.

(a) Native Americans follow these three concepts:

1 Prevention.

2 Treatment.

3 Health maintenance.

(b) The person's health is defined in terms of the person's relationship with nature and the universe.

b. **Examples of Differences in Treatment of Disorders**.

(1) Blacks and Raza/Latino cultures have long used roots, potions, and herbs for treating illnesses.

(2) Filipinos and Raza/Latino groups believe that:

(a) Hotness and coldness, wetness and dryness, must be balanced to be healthy.

(b) Certain illnesses are hot or cold, wet or dry.

(c) Certain foods and medications, classified as hot or cold, are added or subtracted to bring about a balance of humors or to fight off "hot" or "cold" illnesses.

(3) Copper bracelets are worn by some groups as a preventive or cure for arthritis.

c. **Other Cultural Influences to Consider When Planning Nursing Care**.

(1) The nurse should take into consideration the needs of people who practice folk healing. The folk healer (curandero in Spanish) should be allowed to see the patient.

(2) South Americans often wear chains to drive away evil spirits. The nurse should not remove these unless it is absolutely necessary.

(3) Native American women are not likely to seek early prenatal care. They believe that pregnancy is a natural, normal process; a clinic or a hospital is associated with illness.

(4) Many Latino patients believe that it is dangerous to bathe immediately after delivery. The nurse must remember this during postpartum care.

(5) Many cultural groups, such as Native Americans and Southeast Asians, believe that it is improper or impolite to look someone in the eye when speaking to him/her.

## 1-31. RELIGIOUS BELIEFS ABOUT ILLNESS AND DEATH

a. **The Jewish Religion**.

(1) Practices.

(a) Dietary practices vary among Orthodox, Conservative, and Reform Jews.

1 The patient should be asked if/how he/she observes the Kosher dietary laws.

2 The head nurse or dietician should be notified so that the dietary practices can be considered when meals are prepared and served.

(b) The Jewish person is expected by the culture to be independent and self-reliant; and emphasis is placed upon responsibilities and obligations to God.

(c) All practicing Jews observe Saturday as the Sabbath.

(d) The most important Jewish holidays are Yom Kippur, Rosh Hashanah, and Passover.

(e) The patient may wish to see the Rabbi (spiritual leader).

(f) Circumcision of male infants is generally a religious ceremony and is sometimes performed at the hospital.

(2) Nursing implications.

(a) Although it is usually not possible to serve Kosher meat in a nonsectarian hospital, the nurse can be sure not to serve meat and dairy foods together or pork to an Orthodox Jewish patient.

(b) Allow the patient to be as independent as possible and make as many of his/her own decisions as possible.

(c) Be especially observant for indications that a patient needs pain medications because he/she may not tell you if he/she needs them. These indications may be:

1 Restlessness.

2 Diaphoresis (perspiration, often perfuse).

3 A distressed facial expression.

4 Withdrawal.

(d) You may have to help arrange for a place in the hospital to have a male child circumcised.

(e) Arrange for a Rabbi to visit the patient on Saturdays or special holidays.

b. **The Protestant Faith**.

(1) Practices.

(a) There are many denominations in the Protestant faith. Most denominations recognize two sacraments: Baptism and Communion.

(b) A person may be baptized by a layperson, such as a nurse, in an emergency.

(c) Christmas and Easter are the most important Christian holidays for Protestants, as for other Christians.

(2) Nursing implications.

(a) Ask the patient if he/she would like a visit from a Minister or other member of the church.

(b) In the event of an emergency in which an infant or adult may become critical and/or die, the nurse may baptize the patient, if asked, or may do it if he/she (the nurse) thinks it may be comforting to the patient and/or family.

(c) Inquire about any specific dietary or religious practices and provide this information to the appropriate person.

c. **The Roman Catholic Faith.**

(1) Practices.

(a) The Roman Catholic Church considers Baptism, Confession, Holy Communion, and the Sacrament of the Sick as basic sacraments of the Church.

(b) During a long illness, a Catholic patient usually wants a priest to hear confession and to give communion. At such times, the nurse should provide as much privacy as possible.

(c) Death is viewed from three aspects:

1 Visible reaction: emphasis on faith in God.

2 Fear of dying and of judgment: trying to get life in order.

3 Desire for death: emphasis on returning to God.

(d) The last rites of the Church (Sacrament of the Sick)

1 A vital part of the Catholic faith.

2 Comforts both the patient and the family members.

(e) Easter and Christmas are the most important holidays in the Roman Catholic faith.

(f) Many Catholics abstain from or restrict their intake of meat during Lent, which is the 40-day period from Ash Wednesday to Easter. Some have maintained the custom of abstaining from meat on Fridays.

(2) Nursing implications.

(a) In case of an emergency or impending death, a member of the nursing staff may perform a Baptism.

(b) If a patient is brought into the hospital unconscious or in a serious condition and found to have a rosary, Catholic medal, or identification card indicating that the patient is Catholic, a priest should be called so the patient may have the Sacrament of the Sick.

(3) If a patient wishes to abstain from meat because of a religious holiday, inform the dietician or head nurse so that arrangements can be made.

(4) During important holidays, the patient may want to see a priest and/or attend Mass.

d. **Christian Science**.

(1) Practices.

(a) Christian Scientists do not permit surgery or many other forms of medical care.

(b) They believe that all illness is mental in origin.

(c) They believe that illness can be cured by appropriate mental processes.

(d) Treatment consists of prayer and counsel for the sick person; healing is carried out by certified practitioners.

(e) Healing is highly intellectual.

(f) There is no formal clergy.

(2) Nursing implications.

(a) Because surgery or other medical care is not permitted, often legal intervention must be obtained in order to give care in an emergency situation.

(b) Because there is no formal clergy, arrangements may have to be made to have other church members visit the patient.

e. **The Latter Day Saints**.

(1) Practices.

(a) Mormons are members of the Church of Jesus Christ of Latter Day Saints.

(b) They believe in the laying on of hands in treating deformities.

(c) They do not use tobacco; drink stimulants (such as coffee, tea, or cola drinks) or alcoholic beverages; or consume chocolate.

(2) Nursing implications.

(a) Inform the dietician or Head Nurse of the patient's dietary requirements.

(b) Ask the patient if he/she has any particular religious practices he/she wishes to follow and adhere to them if possible.

***Continue with Exercises***

**EXERCISES, LESSON 1**

**INSTRUCTIONS.** The following exercises are to be answered by completing the incomplete statement or by writing the answer in the space provided at the end of the question.

After you have completed all the exercises, turn to "Solutions to Exercises" at the end of the lesson and check your answers.

1. Health can be defined as a state of complete physical, mental, and ______________________ well-being, not merely the absence of disease or ____________________________________________________________.

2. Total health includes the following aspects:

   a. ________________________ health.

   b. ________________________ health.

   c. ________________________health.

   d. ________________________ health.

3. An individual experiences various states of health and illness that fluctuate throughout his life. This is referred to as the health-illness _________________.

4. It is our ____________________or ________________________ to change (rather than the change itself) that affects our health.

5. The individual's state of health is determined by the ability to adapt to changes in which dimensions?

   a. ___________________________________________

   b. ___________________________________________

   c. ___________________________________________

   d. ___________________________________________

6. What are the three main categories of basic human needs?

a. ____________________ needs.

b. ____________________ needs.

c. ____________________ needs

7. Name three physical needs.

a. ____________________________________________

b. ____________________________________________

c. ____________________________________________

8. Name two emotional needs.

a. ______________________________________

b. ______________________________________

9. Name two social needs.

a. ______________________________________

b. ______________________________________

10. Name the six categories contained in Maslow's Hierarchy of Needs.

a. ________________________________________

b. ________________________________________

c. ________________________________________

d. ________________________________________

e. ________________________________________

f. ________________________________________

11. The major purpose of communication is to send, receive, interpret, and _____________ appropriately and clearly to a message, an __________________ of information.

12. The means of transmitting an idea is called the _________________

13. The response to a message is called ____________

14. Rapport is the harmonious feeling experienced by two people who hold one another in mutual respect, acceptance, and ________________

15. If you must ask a patient a personal or embarrassing question, explain _______ and keep it short and matter-of-fact.

16. When speaking to a patient, is it best to sit or stand? __________________

17. If you have three questions to ask your patient, is it better to ask all three of the questions and then let him answer or to ask him one question at a time? ______________________________.

18. If you use the technique of reflection during an interview, you might reflect on what the patient has actually said or on what you think the patient is ______________.

19. An occasional brief response during an interview, such as a nod of the head or saying "I see" is called________________________.

20. If you find that your needs conflict with those of your patient's, what should you do? _________________________________________________________.

21. When you enter the room of a patient who is blind, what is the first thing you should do? ____________________________________________________.

22. Before touching a patient who is blind, be sure to _____________________

23. Do not cover your mouth when you are speaking with a patient who is deaf because he/she may ___________________.

24. If you need a translator in order to communicate with a patient who speaks a foreign language, you may find assistance at ______________________or ____________________________.

25. Name two factors, which influence whether a person will seek or avoid professional help.

a. ____________________________________________________.

b. ____________________________________________________.

26. Name three factors, which cause stress to hospitalized patients.

a. ____________________________________________________.

b. ____________________________________________________.

c. ____________________________________________________.

27. In the first stage of illness, the patient may refuse to get the care, which he needs. What is the name of this stage? ____________________________________

28. In the second stage of illness, the patient focuses his attention on his symptoms and his illness and often feels dependent on health care personnel. What is this stage called? ________________________

29. In the third and final stage of illness, the patient "learns to live with" his perceived loss or impairment of function. What is the name of this stage of illness?

______________________________________________________

30. Name three common emotional reactions to illness and hospitalization.

______________________________

______________________________

______________________________

31. What is the term used to describe a state of alertness and readiness for action in order to avoid or escape harm? ______________________________

32. Does a person experiencing anxiety generally know why he is feeling anxious?

______________________________

33. Name four common physiologic symptoms of anxiety.

______________________________

______________________________

______________________________

______________________________

34. Stress may be experienced as a result of a situation, which requires an increased, and often ____________________ effort to adjust.

35. If you are facing an unpleasant experience, and there is nothing you can do to change the situation, you may experience feelings of ____________________.

36. What is one thing that all aspects of trans-cultural nursing must have in common?

______________________________

37. Name two disorders, which are specific to cultural groups.

a. ____________________.

b. ____________________.

38. A traditional belief of the Japanese Shintoist is that illness is a result of contact with __________________________________________.

39. Native Americans view a person's health in terms of his relationship with nature and the ____________________________

40. What is the name of the 40-day period (from Ash Wednesday to Easter) in which many Catholics abstain from or restrict their intake of meat?

__________________________________

***Check Your Answers on Next Page***

**SOLUTIONS TO EXERCISES, LESSON 1**

1. Social, infirmity. (para 1-2a(2))

2. Social.
   Mental.
   Emotional.
   Spiritual. (paras 1-2b(1)--(4))

3. Continuum. (para 1-3a)

4. Adaptation, response. (para 1-3b)

5. Developmental.
   Psychosocial.
   Cultural.
   Physiological. (paras 1-4a--d)

6. Physical.
   Emotional.
   Social. (paras 1-6a--c)

7. A correct answer consists of any three of the following:

   Food.
   Water.
   Oxygen.
   Elimination.
   Clothing and shelter.
   Activity or sensory and motor stimulation. (paras 1-6a(1)--6))

8. A correct answer consists of any two of the following:

   Love.
   Importance.
   Adequacy.
   Productivity. (paras 1-6b(1)--(4))

9. A correct answer consists of any two of the following:

   Identification or belonging.
   Education or learning.
   Recreation or play.
   Religion or worship. (paras 1-6c(1)--(4))

10. Physiological.
    Safety.
    Love and belonging.
    Esteem and recognition.
    Self-actualization.
    Aesthetic. (paras 1-7a(1)--(6))

11. Respond, interchange. (para 1-11a)

12. Channel. (para 1-12c)

13. Feedback. (para 1-12e)

14. Undertaking. (para 1-14a)

15. Why. (para 1-15b(1))

16. Sit. (para 1-16a(3))

17. One question at a time. (para 1-16b(4))

18. Feeling. (para 1-16c(1))

19. Facilitation. (para 1-16c(3))

20. Find sources other than the therapeutic relationship to meet your own needs. (para 1-18c)

21. Speak to the patient so he will know who is there. (para 1-19a(1))

22. Speak to the patient. (para 1-19a(4))

23. Read lips. (para 1-19b(2))

24. The Red Cross or the Patient Administration Division (PAD). (para 1-19c(1))

25. A correct answer consists of any two of the following:

    The degree and extent of symptom distress.
    Expectation of return to health if treatment is instituted.
    Fear of diagnostic and treatment procedures.
    Fear of discovery of serious illness.
    The self-concept that one is always healthy. (paras 1-22a--e)

26. A correct answer consists of any three of the following:

    Unfamiliarity of surroundings.
    Loss of independence.
    Separation from spouse.
    Separation from family.
    Financial problems.
    Isolation from other people.
    Lack of information.
    Threat of severe illness.
    Problems with medications. (paras 1-23a--i)

27. Denial (or disbelief in being ill). (para 1-24a)

28. Acceptance (of being ill). (para 1-24b)

29. Recovery, rehabilitation, or convalescence. (para 1-24c)

30. A correct answer consists of any three of the following:

    Fear.
    Anxiety.
    Stress.
    Over dependency or feelings of helplessness. (para 1-25)

31. "Fight or flight" reaction. (para 1-25a(4)(f))

32. No. (para 1-25b(2))

33. A correct answer consists of any four of the following:

    Fatigue.
    Insomnia.
    Diarrhea or constipation.
    Urgency.
    Nausea.
    Anorexia.
    Excessive perspiration. (paras 1-25b(4)(a)--(g))

34. Prolonged. (para 1-25c(2))

35. Helplessness. (para 1-25d(2))

36. Respect for the patient. (para 1-27)

37. Tay-Sachs and sickle cell anemia. (para 1-29s)

38. Pollutants (such as blood or a corpse). (para 1-30a(1)(b))

39. Universe. (para 1-30a(2)(b))

40. Lent. (para 1-31c(1)(f))

***END OF LESSON 1***

## LESSON ASSIGNMENT

**LESSON 2** The Adult Patient Care Unit.

**TEXT ASSIGNMENT** Paragraphs 2-1 through 2-7.

**LESSON OBJECTIVES** After completing this lesson, you should be able to:

2-1. Identify items of furniture normally found in the patient care area.

2-2. Identify articles/equipment required in the patient care area.

2-3. Identify guidelines/methods of bed-making.

2-4. Identify guidelines for terminally cleaning the patient care unit.

2-5. Recognize rules for the use of disposable and non-disposable items.

**SUGGESTION** After studying the assignment, complete the exercises at the end of this lesson. These exercises will help you to achieve the lesson objectives.

## LESSON 2

## THE ADULT PATIENT CARE UNIT

### 2-1. INTRODUCTION

The patient care unit is the area of the hospital in which the patient receives medical and nursing care and treatment as well as the place in which he/she lives during his/her hospital stay. It must be maintained as a safe, pleasant, clean, and orderly environment for the patient's physical and mental well being. Constant effort is needed to achieve and maintain the necessary high level of order and sanitation.

### 2-2. FURNITURE COMPRISING THE PATIENT BASIC UNIT

Furniture for the patient basic unit includes:

a. Bed.

b. Bedside cabinet.

c. Overbed table.

d. Chair.

### 2-3. EQUIPMENT/ARTICLES NECESSARY FOR PROVIDING BASIC NURSING CARE

The following are provided to the patient:

a. **Linens**.

(1) Bed linens.

(2) Towels.

(3) Washcloths.

(4) Blankets.

b. **Toilet Equipment.**

(1) Wash basin.

(2) Soap dish.

(3) Emesis basin.

(4) Bedpan.

(5) Urinal.

(6) Toilet paper.

c. **Other Articles.**

(1) Water pitcher.

(2) Glass.

(3) Call button.

(4) Disposable facial tissues.

## 2-4. GUIDELINES FOR BED-MAKING

a. Gather all the required linen and accessories before making the bed.

(1) Sheets.

(2) Pillowcases.

(3) Blankets.

(4) Bedspread.

(5) Extra pillows.

b. Avoid shaking the linen to prevent the spread of microorganisms and dust particles.

c. Avoid placing linens, clean or dirty, on another patient's bed.

d. Do not place dirty linen on the floor.

e. Do not hold dirty linen against your uniform.

f. Always use good body mechanics; raise the bed to its highest position to make bed-making easier.

g. Stay on one side of the bed until it is completely made; then move to the other side and finish the bed. This saves time and steps.

h. Observe the patient and document any nursing observations.

(1) Check for areas of redness that may lead to decubiti formation.

(2) Note tolerance of activity level while out of bed.

(3) Note observations about the physical and emotional status of the patient.

(4) Note any patient teaching or reinforced teaching given and the patient's response.

(5) Check for drainage, wetness, or other body fluids and record observations.

## 2-5. METHODS OF BED-MAKING

a. **Unoccupied (Closed) Bed**. An unoccupied bed is one that is made when not occupied by a patient.

(1) Raise the bed to a comfortable working height, if adjustable.

(2) Lower siderails, if present.

(3) Remove pillows and pillowcases. Set the pillows aside in a clean area.

(4) Fold and set the blankets and spreads aside (to be reused).

(5) Loosen the linen along the edges of the bed, and move toward the end of the bed.

(6) Wash the mattress if necessary, turn the mattress to the opposite side if necessary, and replace the mattress pad as needed. Observe the mattress for protruding springs.

(7) Place the bottom sheet.

(a) Flat sheet.

1 Position evenly on the bed.

2 Miter the corners at the top of the bed. Lift the mattress slightly, then stretch and tie the ends of the sheet together beneath the mattress. Repeat these steps for the bottom of the bed.

3 Stretch and tuck the free edges at the sides.

(b) Fitted sheet.

1 Fit the sheet on the lower edges of the mattress first. Then lift the mattress and fit the sheet on the top edges of the mattress.

2 Stretch and tuck the free edges at the sides.

(8) Place a draw sheet on the center of the bed, if it is needed.

(a) Tuck in the free edge on one side.

(b) Stretch the draw sheet from the opposite side and tuck in the free edge.

(9) Place the top sheet, blanket (if used), and bedspread.

(a) Position evenly on the bed.

(b) Miter the bottom corners, tucking all three parts together.

(c) Leave the loose ends free.

(10) Fanfold the top linen back to the foot of the bed.

(11) Place a clean pillowcase over the pillow and place it at the head of the bed.

(a) Invert the pillowcase over one hand so the inner back seam is visible.

(b) Grasp the edge of the pillow with one hand holding the pillowcase at the seam.

(c) Use the opposite hand to guide the pillowcase over the pillow.

(12) Adjust the bed to its lowest position, if adjustable.

(13) Reposition the head up slightly, if the patient prefers.

(14) Raise the siderail opposite the side of the bed where the patient will enter.

b. **Occupied (Open) Bed**. An occupied bed is one that is made while occupied by a patient.

(1) Wash your hands.

(2) Identify the patient, explain the procedure, and be sure you will have the patient's cooperation.

(3) Check the condition of the bed linens to determine which supplies you will need.

(4) Provide for the patient's privacy (throughout the procedure).

(5) Obtain the articles of linen that you will need.

(6) Place the bath blanket over the patient and the top cover.

(7) Loosen the top bedding from the foot of the bed and remove it. If possible, have the patient hold the bath blanket while you pull the top covers from under it from the foot of the bed.

(8) Move the mattress to the head of the bed.

(9) Move the patient to the distal side of the bed.

(10) Make the bed on one side.

(11) Move or turn the patient to the clean side of the bed, and finish making the bed on the opposite side. Place the clean linen on top, and remove the bath blanket.

(12) Attach the patient's signal cord within reach.

(13) Provide for the patient's safety and comfort.

(14) Tidy the room.

c. **Anesthetic, Surgical, or Post-Op Bed**. This is a bed that is prepared to receive a patient from the operating room.

(1) Gather all needed supplies:

(a) Large sheets (2).

(b) Drawsheet (1) or an additional large sheet.

(c) Blanket.

(d) Pillow(s).

(e) Pillowcase(s).

(f) Towel.

(g) Chux®, if drainage is anticipated.

(2) Make the bed as though you are making an unoccupied bed, except that the top sheet and blanket are not tucked under the mattress at the foot of the bed, and the corners are not mitered.

(3) Fanfold the top covers to the side or to the foot of the bed.

(4) Place a towel or disposable pad (Chux®) at the head of the bed. This is intended to protect the sheet if the patient should vomit.

(5) It is a good idea to place a drawsheet on the bed because it can be used to move the patient more easily.

(6) Place the pillow(s) on a chair near the bed or in an upright position at the head of the bed.

(7) Leave the bed in the high position.

(8) Lock the brakes on the bed.

(9) Move the furniture away from the bed to allow for easier access to the bed for the recovery room stretcher and personnel.

(10) Make certain an emesis basin is readily available and suction is available where indicated.

(11) Keep Chux® available to use if necessary.

## 2-6. TERMINAL CLEANING OF THE PATIENT CARE UNIT

a. **Definition**.

(1) The sanitation of the bed, bedside cabinet, and general area of the patient care unit with a detergent/germicidal agent after the patient is discharged or transferred from the nursing care unit.

(2) Performed at every patient care unit before the area is prepared for the next patient.

b. **Reasons for Terminal Cleaning of the Patient Care Unit**.

(1) Prevention of the spread of microorganisms.

(2) Removal of encrusted secretions from framework or bedside rails.

(3) Removal of residue of body wastes from the mattress.

(4) Deodorizing of the bed frame, mattress, and pillow.

c. **Guidelines for Terminal Cleaning.**

(1) Review ward SOP for specific procedures.

(2) Use only authorized disinfectant/detergent or germicidal solution for cleaning.

(3) Check to ensure the bedside cabinet is cleared of any valuables belonging to the patient.

(4) Check bed linens for personal items (dentures, contact lenses, money, jewelry, etc.) belonging to the patient.

(5) Prevent spread of microorganisms by carefully removing linen from the bed.

(6) Use caution when cleaning the underframe and bedsprings.

(7) Replace any torn mattress or pillow covers.

(8) Allow the mattress and pillow to air-dry thoroughly before remaking the bed.

## 2-7. RULES FOR USE OF DISPOSABLE OR NONREUSABLE ITEMS

a. Do not attempt to reuse (for another patient) or resterilize disposables.

b. Sterile disposables are considered sterile providing the wrapper is not broken or torn or the expiration date has not passed.

c. Sterile disposables with torn or broken wrappers must be discarded.

d. Use disposables for the specific purpose(s) for which they were designed.

e. Follow manufacturer's directions when using disposables.

Continue with Exercises

## EXERCISES, LESSON 2

**INSTRUCTIONS.** The following exercises are to be answered by completing the incomplete statement or by writing the answer in the space provided at the end of the question.

After you have completed all the exercises, turn to "Solutions to Exercises" at the end of the lesson and check your answers.

1. Name the four items of furniture comprising the patient basic unit.

   a. ____________________________.

   b. ____________________________.

   c. ____________________________.

   d. ____________________________.

2. Name three items, other than linens and toilet equipment, which the patient is given.

   a. ____________________________.

   b. ____________________________.

   c. ____________________________.

3. When making a bed, avoid shaking the linen to prevent spread of ________________________ and dust particles.

4. When making a bed, always raise the bed to its ________________ position.

5. When making a bed, check the patient for areas of redness that may lead to ____________________ formation.

6. When making an unoccupied bed, be sure to check the mattress for protruding ____________________.

7. Before removing the top bedding from an occupied bed, place the ___________________________ over the patient and the top cover.

8. When making a surgical bed, do you tuck the top sheet and blanket under the mattress at the foot of the bed? ______

9. To protect the sheets, place a towel or disposable pad (Chux ®) at the ________ of a surgical bed.

10. After making a surgical bed, be sure to lock the _________________.

11. When a patient is discharged or transferred out of the patient care unit, the bed, bedside cabinet, and general area must be sanitized with a detergent/germicidal agent. What is this procedure called? _______________________________.

12. Name three reasons for terminal cleaning of the patient care unit.

    a. _________________________________________________________________.

    b. _________________________________________________________________.

    c. _________________________________________________________________.

13. During terminal cleaning, use only ____________________ disinfectant/detergent or germicidal solution.

14. How should you prevent the spread of microorganisms during terminal cleaning?

    _________________________________________________________________.

15. Sterile disposables are considered sterile if the wrapper is not broken or torn or if the _____________________________ has not passed.

***Check Your Answers on Next Page***

**SOLUTIONS TO EXERCISES, LESSON 2**

1. Bed
   Bedside cabinet
   Overbed table
   Chair (paras 2-2a--d)

2. A correct answer consists of any three of the following:

   Water pitcher
   Glass
   Call button
   Disposable facial tissues (paras 2-3c(1)--(4))

3. Microorganisms (para 2-4b)

4. Highest (para 2-4f)

5. Decubiti (para 2-4h(1))

6. Springs (para 2-5a(6))

7. Bath blanket (para 2-5b(6))

8. No (para 2-5c(2))

9. Head (para 2-5c(4))

10. Brakes (para 2-5c(8))

11. Terminal cleaning (para 2-6a(1))

12. A correct answer consists of any three of the following:

    Prevention of the spread of microorganisms
    Removal of encrusted secretions from framework or bedside rails
    Removal of residue of body wastes from the mattress
    Deodorizing of the bedframe, mattress, and pillow (paras 2-6b(1)--(4))

13. Authorized (para 2-6c(2))

14. By carefully removing linen from the bed (para 2-6c(5))

15. Expiration date (para 2-7b)

*Return to Table of Contents*

## LESSON ASSIGNMENT

**LESSON 2** The Adult Patient Care Unit.

**TEXT ASSIGNMENT** Paragraphs 2-1 through 2-7.

**LESSON OBJECTIVES** After completing this lesson, you should be able to:

2-1. Identify items of furniture normally found in the patient care area.

2-2. Identify articles/equipment required in the patient care area.

2-3. Identify guidelines/methods of bed-making.

2-4. Identify guidelines for terminally cleaning the patient care unit.

2-5. Recognize rules for the use of disposable and non-disposable items.

**SUGGESTION** After studying the assignment, complete the exercises at the end of this lesson. These exercises will help you to achieve the lesson objectives.

# LESSON 2

# THE ADULT PATIENT CARE UNIT

## 2-1. INTRODUCTION

The patient care unit is the area of the hospital in which the patient receives medical and nursing care and treatment as well as the place in which he/she lives during his/her hospital stay. It must be maintained as a safe, pleasant, clean, and orderly environment for the patient's physical and mental well being. Constant effort is needed to achieve and maintain the necessary high level of order and sanitation.

## 2-2. FURNITURE COMPRISING THE PATIENT BASIC UNIT

Furniture for the patient basic unit includes:

a. Bed.

b. Bedside cabinet.

c. Overbed table.

d. Chair.

## 2-3. EQUIPMENT/ARTICLES NECESSARY FOR PROVIDING BASIC NURSING CARE

The following are provided to the patient:

a. **Linens**.

(1) Bed linens.

(2) Towels.

(3) Washcloths.

(4) Blankets.

b. **Toilet Equipment.**

(1) Wash basin.

(2) Soap dish.

(3) Emesis basin.

(4) Bedpan.

(5) Urinal.

(6) Toilet paper.

c. **Other Articles.**

(1) Water pitcher.

(2) Glass.

(3) Call button.

(4) Disposable facial tissues.

## 2-4. GUIDELINES FOR BED-MAKING

a. Gather all the required linen and accessories before making the bed.

(1) Sheets.

(2) Pillowcases.

(3) Blankets.

(4) Bedspread.

(5) Extra pillows.

b. Avoid shaking the linen to prevent the spread of microorganisms and dust particles.

c. Avoid placing linens, clean or dirty, on another patient's bed.

d. Do not place dirty linen on the floor.

e. Do not hold dirty linen against your uniform.

f. Always use good body mechanics; raise the bed to its highest position to make bed-making easier.

g. Stay on one side of the bed until it is completely made; then move to the other side and finish the bed. This saves time and steps.

h. Observe the patient and document any nursing observations.

(1) Check for areas of redness that may lead to decubiti formation.

(2) Note tolerance of activity level while out of bed.

(3) Note observations about the physical and emotional status of the patient.

(4) Note any patient teaching or reinforced teaching given and the patient's response.

(5) Check for drainage, wetness, or other body fluids and record observations.

## 2-5. METHODS OF BED-MAKING

a. **Unoccupied (Closed) Bed**. An unoccupied bed is one that is made when not occupied by a patient.

(1) Raise the bed to a comfortable working height, if adjustable.

(2) Lower siderails, if present.

(3) Remove pillows and pillowcases. Set the pillows aside in a clean area.

(4) Fold and set the blankets and spreads aside (to be reused).

(5) Loosen the linen along the edges of the bed, and move toward the end of the bed.

(6) Wash the mattress if necessary, turn the mattress to the opposite side if necessary, and replace the mattress pad as needed. Observe the mattress for protruding springs.

(7) Place the bottom sheet.

(a) Flat sheet.

<u>1</u> Position evenly on the bed.

2 Miter the corners at the top of the bed. Lift the mattress slightly, then stretch and tie the ends of the sheet together beneath the mattress. Repeat these steps for the bottom of the bed.

3 Stretch and tuck the free edges at the sides.

(b) Fitted sheet.

1 Fit the sheet on the lower edges of the mattress first. Then lift the mattress and fit the sheet on the top edges of the mattress.

2 Stretch and tuck the free edges at the sides.

(8) Place a draw sheet on the center of the bed, if it is needed.

(a) Tuck in the free edge on one side.

(b) Stretch the draw sheet from the opposite side and tuck in the free edge.

(9) Place the top sheet, blanket (if used), and bedspread.

(a) Position evenly on the bed.

(b) Miter the bottom corners, tucking all three parts together.

(c) Leave the loose ends free.

(10) Fanfold the top linen back to the foot of the bed.

(11) Place a clean pillowcase over the pillow and place it at the head of the bed.

(a) Invert the pillowcase over one hand so the inner back seam is visible.

(b) Grasp the edge of the pillow with one hand holding the pillowcase at the seam.

(c) Use the opposite hand to guide the pillowcase over the pillow.

(12) Adjust the bed to its lowest position, if adjustable.

(13) Reposition the head up slightly, if the patient prefers.

(14) Raise the siderail opposite the side of the bed where the patient will enter.

b. **Occupied (Open) Bed**. An occupied bed is one that is made while occupied by a patient.

(1) Wash your hands.

(2) Identify the patient, explain the procedure, and be sure you will have the patient's cooperation.

(3) Check the condition of the bed linens to determine which supplies you will need.

(4) Provide for the patient's privacy (throughout the procedure).

(5) Obtain the articles of linen that you will need.

(6) Place the bath blanket over the patient and the top cover.

(7) Loosen the top bedding from the foot of the bed and remove it. If possible, have the patient hold the bath blanket while you pull the top covers from under it from the foot of the bed.

(8) Move the mattress to the head of the bed.

(9) Move the patient to the distal side of the bed.

(10) Make the bed on one side.

(11) Move or turn the patient to the clean side of the bed, and finish making the bed on the opposite side. Place the clean linen on top, and remove the bath blanket.

(12) Attach the patient's signal cord within reach.

(13) Provide for the patient's safety and comfort.

(14) Tidy the room.

c. **Anesthetic, Surgical, or Post-Op Bed**. This is a bed that is prepared to receive a patient from the operating room.

(1) Gather all needed supplies:

(a) Large sheets (2).

(b) Drawsheet (1) or an additional large sheet.

(c) Blanket.

(d) Pillow(s).

(e) Pillowcase(s).

(f) Towel.

(g) Chux®, if drainage is anticipated.

(2) Make the bed as though you are making an unoccupied bed, except that the top sheet and blanket are not tucked under the mattress at the foot of the bed, and the corners are not mitered.

(3) Fanfold the top covers to the side or to the foot of the bed.

(4) Place a towel or disposable pad (Chux®) at the head of the bed. This is intended to protect the sheet if the patient should vomit.

(5) It is a good idea to place a drawsheet on the bed because it can be used to move the patient more easily.

(6) Place the pillow(s) on a chair near the bed or in an upright position at the head of the bed.

(7) Leave the bed in the high position.

(8) Lock the brakes on the bed.

(9) Move the furniture away from the bed to allow for easier access to the bed for the recovery room stretcher and personnel.

(10) Make certain an emesis basin is readily available and suction is available where indicated.

(11) Keep Chux® available to use if necessary.

## 2-6. TERMINAL CLEANING OF THE PATIENT CARE UNIT

a. **Definition.**

(1) The sanitation of the bed, bedside cabinet, and general area of the patient care unit with a detergent/germicidal agent after the patient is discharged or transferred from the nursing care unit.

(2) Performed at every patient care unit before the area is prepared for the next patient.

b. **Reasons for Terminal Cleaning of the Patient Care Unit**.

(1) Prevention of the spread of microorganisms.

(2) Removal of encrusted secretions from framework or bedside rails.

(3) Removal of residue of body wastes from the mattress.

(4) Deodorizing of the bed frame, mattress, and pillow.

c. **Guidelines for Terminal Cleaning.**

(1) Review ward SOP for specific procedures.

(2) Use only authorized disinfectant/detergent or germicidal solution for cleaning.

(3) Check to ensure the bedside cabinet is cleared of any valuables belonging to the patient.

(4) Check bed linens for personal items (dentures, contact lenses, money, jewelry, etc.) belonging to the patient.

(5) Prevent spread of microorganisms by carefully removing linen from the bed.

(6) Use caution when cleaning the underframe and bedsprings.

(7) Replace any torn mattress or pillow covers.

(8) Allow the mattress and pillow to air-dry thoroughly before remaking the bed.

## 2-7. RULES FOR USE OF DISPOSABLE OR NONREUSABLE ITEMS

a. Do not attempt to reuse (for another patient) or resterilize disposables.

b. Sterile disposables are considered sterile providing the wrapper is not broken or torn or the expiration date has not passed.

c. Sterile disposables with torn or broken wrappers must be discarded.

d. Use disposables for the specific purpose(s) for which they were designed.

e. Follow manufacturer's directions when using disposables.

***Continue with Exercises***

**EXERCISES, LESSON 2**

**INSTRUCTIONS.** The following exercises are to be answered by completing the incomplete statement or by writing the answer in the space provided at the end of the question.

After you have completed all the exercises, turn to "Solutions to Exercises" at the end of the lesson and check your answers.

1. Name the four items of furniture comprising the patient basic unit.

   a. ______________________________.

   b. ______________________________.

   c. ______________________________.

   d. ______________________________.

2. Name three items, other than linens and toilet equipment, which the patient is given.

   a. ______________________________.

   b. ______________________________.

   c. ______________________________.

3. When making a bed, avoid shaking the linen to prevent spread of ________________________ and dust particles.

4. When making a bed, always raise the bed to its ________________ position.

5. When making a bed, check the patient for areas of redness that may lead to ____________________ formation.

6. When making an unoccupied bed, be sure to check the mattress for protruding ________________.

7. Before removing the top bedding from an occupied bed, place the ______________________ over the patient and the top cover.

8. When making a surgical bed, do you tuck the top sheet and blanket under the mattress at the foot of the bed? ______

9. To protect the sheets, place a towel or disposable pad (Chux ®) at the ________ of a surgical bed.

10. After making a surgical bed, be sure to lock the _______________.

11. When a patient is discharged or transferred out of the patient care unit, the bed, bedside cabinet, and general area must be sanitized with a detergent/germicidal agent. What is this procedure called? ___________________________.

12. Name three reasons for terminal cleaning of the patient care unit.

    a. ______________________________________________________.

    b. ______________________________________________________.

    c. ______________________________________________________.

13. During terminal cleaning, use only _________________ disinfectant/detergent or germicidal solution.

14. How should you prevent the spread of microorganisms during terminal cleaning?

    ______________________________________________________.

15. Sterile disposables are considered sterile if the wrapper is not broken or torn or if the ________________________ has not passed.

***Check Your Answers on Next Page***

## SOLUTIONS TO EXERCISES, LESSON 2

1. Bed
   Bedside cabinet
   Overbed table
   Chair (paras 2-2a--d)

2. A correct answer consists of any three of the following:

   Water pitcher
   Glass
   Call button
   Disposable facial tissues (paras 2-3c(1)--(4))

3. Microorganisms (para 2-4b)

4. Highest (para 2-4f)

5. Decubiti (para 2-4h(1))

6. Springs (para 2-5a(6))

7. Bath blanket (para 2-5b(6))

8. No (para 2-5c(2))

9. Head (para 2-5c(4))

10. Brakes (para 2-5c(8))

11. Terminal cleaning (para 2-6a(1))

12. A correct answer consists of any three of the following:

    Prevention of the spread of microorganisms
    Removal of encrusted secretions from framework or bedside rails
    Removal of residue of body wastes from the mattress
    Deodorizing of the bedframe, mattress, and pillow (paras 2-6b(1)--(4))

13. Authorized (para 2-6c(2))

14. By carefully removing linen from the bed (para 2-6c(5))

15. Expiration date (para 2-7b)

***END OF LESSON 2***

## LESSON ASSIGNMENT

**LESSON 3** Advanced Principles of Patient Hygiene.

**LESSON ASSIGNMENT** Paragraphs 3-1 through 3-14.

**LESSON OBJECTIVES** After completing this lesson, you should be able to:

3-1. Determine purposes for giving a patient a bath.

3-2. Identify conditions, which encourage skin breakdown.

3-3. Identify interventions, which can prevent skin breakdown.

3-4. Identify patient needs to consider and observations to make during the bathing procedures.

3-5. Identify the principles of mouth care, to include the patient with dentures, the patient with mouth complications, and the unconscious patient.

3-6. Identify the principles and reasons for the back massage.

3-7. Determine guidelines for shaving a male patient.

3-8. Determine guidelines for performing perineal care.

3-9. Identify principles for and purposes of hair care.

**SUGGESTION** After studying the assignment, complete the exercises at the end of this lesson. These exercises will help you to achieve the lesson objectives.

## LESSON 3

## ADVANCED PRINCIPLES OF PATIENT HYGIENE

### 3-1. INTRODUCTION

Providing for a patient's hygiene is probably the most basic of all nursing care activities, but it is undoubtedly one of the most important. Not only is it a provision for the patient's physical needs; it also contributes immeasurably to the patient's feeling of emotional well-being.

### 3-2. PURPOSE OF THE PATIENT'S DAILY BATH

a. Removal of bacteria from the skin.

(1) Confinement in bed increases perspiration, and bacterial growth is stimulated by moisture.

(2) Skin irritation from hospital bed linens may result in skin breakdown and subsequent infection.

b. Relaxation effect on the patient.

c. Stimulation of blood circulation to the skin, respirations, and elimination.

d. Maintenance of joint mobility.

e. Improvement of the patient's self-image and emotional and mental well-being.

f. Providing the nurse with an opportunity for health teaching and assessment.

g. Providing the nurse with an opportunity to give the patient psychological support.

(1) The process of building rapport may begin during the initial bath.

(2) The bath aids in the development of the therapeutic nurse-patient relationship as the patient has the nurse's undivided attention.

### 3-3. PHYSICAL CONDITIONS WHICH ENCOURAGE SKIN BREAKDOWN IN A PATIENT WHO IS CONFINED TO BED

a. **Immobility.** Continuous pressure over any body part impairs circulation to that part and can cause breakdown and eventual ulcerations.

b. **Incontinence**. If the patient is unable to control the bladder or bowel functions, skin breakdown is likely to occur due to the presence of moisture and bacteria on the skin.

c. **Emaciation**. An emaciated patient may be prone to skin breakdown over bony prominence (heels, elbows, and coccyx).

d. **Obesity**. An obese patient may have many skin folds where perspiration and bacteria may contribute to skin breakdown.

e. **Age-Related Skin Changes**. An older person's skin is very thin and inelastic. The sweat and oil glands are less active. Thin, dry skin is more susceptible to pressure areas and skin breakdown.

f. **Any Disease or Condition that Affects Circulation.** Any disease or condition that affects circulation can encourage skin breakdown in a patient who is confined to bed.

## 3-4. NURSING INTERVENTION TO PREVENT SKIN BREAKDOWN

a. The time of the patient's bath or back massage is the most logical time to thoroughly observe the patient's skin for pressure areas.

b. At the first sign of redness, the area should be washed with soap and water and rubbed with lotion; measures should then be taken to keep the patient off the reddened area.

c. Report any signs of pressure to the charge nurse.

d. Keep sheets under the patient clean, smooth, and tight to help eliminate skin irritation.

e. Ensure adequate nutrition and fluid intake, according to physician's orders.

f. Every effort should be made to keep urine and feces off the patient's skin, washing the skin with soap and water and keeping the buttocks and genital area dry (lotion or powder may be used depending upon the patient's skin type) when the patient is incontinent.

g. Obese patients may need assistance washing and drying areas under skin folds (groin, buttocks, under breasts, and so forth.)

h. For the patient with very dry skin, various bath oils may be added to the bath water.

(1) Soap may be omitted because of its drying effect.

(2) Lotions and oils may be used after the bath.

## 3-5. TIMING OF PATIENT HYGIENE PROCEDURES

A patient's bath may be given at any time, according to the patient's needs, but certain routines are generally followed on a ward.

a. **Morning Care.**

(1) The procedure followed in the morning affects the patient's comfort throughout the day.

(2) Each morning before breakfast, the patient should be assisted to the bathroom, or a bedpan or urinal should be provided, according to the patient's activity level.

(3) The patient is then given the opportunity to wash his/her hands and face and brush his/her teeth. The bed linen is straightened, and the overbed table is cleaned in preparation for the breakfast tray.

(4) After breakfast, the patient has a complete bath (type is dependent upon the patient's condition and mobility), mouth care, a change of clothing, and a back massage.

(5) Bed linens are changed; and the unit is cleaned and straightened to provide a comfortable and safe environment for the patient.

b. **Evening Care.**

(1) The care the patient receives at the end of the day greatly influences the patient's level of relaxation and ability to sleep.

(2) An opportunity is provided for elimination; the patient's hands and face are washed; the teeth are brushed; a back rub is given.

(3) Bed linens are straightened; the patient's unit is straightened to ensure comfort and safety. It is important that there are no items, which the patient could slip on, or fall over, such as chairs or linens, on the floor.

## 3-6. PROVIDING FOR SELECTED PATIENT NEEDS WHILE BATHING A PATIENT

a. **Safety.**

(1) The bed may be in the high position during the patient's bed bath, but should be placed in the low position upon completion.

(2) The side rails should be up after the patient's bath for the patient who is confined to the bed.

(a) Side rails help to prevent falls for the elderly patient or the patient who is confused or has a decreased level of consciousness.

(b) The legal aspect requires diligence on the part of nursing personnel.

(3) The patient's call light should be within easy reach to prevent the need to reach for it and risk falling out of bed and to provide easy access in case of pain or distress.

(4) Fire safety in the patient care area calls for the following rules:

(a) No smoking in bed.

(b) No smoking if oxygen is in use.

(5) Always wash your hands before entering and upon leaving the patient's room.

b. **Privacy**.

(1) Respect for the patient's privacy decreases the patient's emotional discomfort during personal care.

(2) Keep the door to the patient's room closed.

(3) Pull the curtains around the unit and drape the patient's body during care.

(4) Allow the patient to complete as much personal care as possible; self-care is appropriate and provides additional privacy.

c. **Comfort**.

(1) Ensure a comfortable temperature in the patient's room.

(2) Close any windows and the door to the patient's room to prevent drafts and chilling.

(3) Drape the patient appropriately during the bath.

(4) For a bedside bath, maintain bath water between 110oF and 115oF; change the water as it cools and/or gets soapy.

## 3-7. SIGNIFICANT NURSING OBSERVATIONS DURING THE BATHING PROCEDURE

a. **Physical Observations**.

(1) Observe the skin under good, natural light.

(2) Any abnormal skin condition should be described as to its location, color, and size and how it feels to the patient.

(3) The following skin observations should be checked upon admission and daily thereafter:

(a) Cleanliness.

(b) Odor. May be caused by sweat secreted by the sweat glands; by abnormal conditions, such as infection or kidney disease; or by bodily discharges (urine, feces) that need to be cleaned.

(c) Texture. Smooth and elastic or dry and rough; nutritional deficiencies can influence skin texture.

(d) Color. Reddened areas that could indicate pressure, cyanosis (bluish tinge) or jaundice (yellowish tinge).

(e) Temperature. Hot skin could mean fever; cold skin could mean poor circulation.

(f) Sensitivity. Pain, tenderness, itching, or burning.

(g) Swelling (edema). Stretched or tight appearing; usually begins in the ankles or legs or any other dependent part; may be associated with injury.

(h) Skin lesions. Rashes, growths, or breaks in the skin.

(4) Observations may begin at the head (scalp) and proceed to the feet in a systematic manner.

b. **Psychosocial Observations**.

(1) Problems in this area may be related to the patient's present problems.

(2) The time of the patient's bath may be a good time to find out more about the patient's psychosocial needs.

(3) Remember that the patient's nonverbal communication may tell you much about the way he/she is feeling.

## 3-8. BASIC PRINCIPLES OF MOUTH CARE

a. **Purposes**.

(1) Provide oral care of the teeth, gums, and mouth.

(2) Remove offensive odors and food debris.

(3) Promote patient comfort and a feeling of well-being.

(4) Preserve the integrity and hydration of the oral mucosa and lips.

(5) Alleviate pain and discomfort, thereby enhancing oral intake.

b. **General Guidelines**.

(1) Oral hygiene should be performed before breakfast, after each meal, and at bedtime.

(2) Oral hygiene is especially important for patients receiving oxygen therapy, patients who have nasogastric tubes, and patients who are NPO. Their oral mucosa dries out much faster than normal due to their mouth-breathing.

(3) You should provide for patient privacy during the procedure, as this is an extremely personal procedure for most patients.

(4) Oral care for the unconscious patient should be performed at least every four hours.

(5) Lipstick, chap stick, or vaseline may be applied to the lips to keep them from drying out.

c. **Nursing Records**. Nursing observations for the patient's mouth should be recorded in the clinical record, noting such factors as:

(1) Bleeding.

(2) Swelling of gums.

(3) Unusual mouth odor.

(4) Effect of brushing the teeth. Note if there is bleeding when you brush the patient's gums and teeth.

d. **Conscious Patients with Dentures**.

(1) General considerations.

(a) Many patients are sensitive or embarrassed about wearing dentures; therefore, the patient's privacy should be respected when the dentures are cleaned.

(b) Dentures must be handled carefully; they are fragile and expensive, and the patient is handicapped without them.

(c) If the dentures are left out of the mouth for any period of time, place them in a covered opaque container with the patient's name on the container.

(d) Dentures must be kept in water to preserve their fit and general quality; the color may change if they become dry.

(e) You may avoid breaking the dentures while cleaning them by holding them over a basin of water with a washcloth folded in the bottom.

(2) Dentures are brushed in the same way as natural teeth; be sure to rinse them well.

(3) The denture cup should be labeled with the patient's name and room number.

(4) Never use hot water to rinse the dentures as it could warp them; use cool or lukewarm water.

(5) The patient's gums and soft tissues should be cared for at least twice per day while the dentures are out of the mouth; a soft-bristled toothbrush, swab, or gauze-covered tongue blade dipped in mouthwash should be used to cleanse the gums, tongue, and soft tissues.

e. **Patients With Mouth Complications.** The following problems are common in patients receiving chemotherapy and radiation therapy:

(1) Bleeding.

(a) Observe the patient's mouth frequently for the amount of bleeding present and the specific areas.

(b) Do not floss the patient's teeth; use a Water-pik®.

(c) Brush the teeth and clean the mouth using one of the following methods:

1 Brush the teeth carefully with a very soft toothbrush.

2 Wrap a tongue blade with a gauze sponge saturated with a prescribed solution; carefully swab the teeth and mouth. Do not use lemon/glycerine swabs or commercial mouthwash because they contain alcohol, which causes burning.

(2) Infection.

(a) Observe the patient's mouth for appearance, integrity, and general condition.

(b) Wear clean gloves during the procedure.

(c) Obtain a culture, if ordered.

(d) Do not floss the teeth if the mouth is irritated or painful.

(e) Assist the patient with brushing the teeth and cleaning the mouth, using a soft toothbrush or a gauze-padded tongue blade.

(f) Rinse the mouth with water and the prescribed solution, if ordered.

(3) Ulcerations, to include stomatitis.

(a) Basic procedure for the patient with an infection should be followed.

(b) If the patient's mouth is extremely painful, rinsing the mouth with a local anesthetic, as prescribed by a physician, may be necessary.

(c) Mouthwash and other solutions which contain alcohol should not be used for the patient with ulcerations as they are frequently very painful.

f. **Unconscious Patients**.

(1) Oral care should be performed at least every four hours.

(2) Oral suctioning may be required for the unconscious patient to prevent aspiration.

(3) A soft toothbrush or gauze-padded tongue blade may be used to clean the teeth and mouth.

(4) The patient should be positioned in the lateral position with the head turned toward the side to provide for drainage and to prevent aspiration.

## 3-9. BACK MASSAGE AS A PATIENT COMFORT MEASURE

a. Decreases muscle tension and promotes relaxation.

b. Increases circulation to the area.

c. Aids in the development of the therapeutic nurse-patient relationship.

## 3-10. BASIC PRINCIPLES OF BACK MASSAGE

a. The psychological benefits of back massage cannot be overstressed for the hospitalized patient.

b. The following statements illustrate the concept of therapeutic touch as an integral part of the domain of nursing.

(1) Touch can be perceived as a manifestation of caring and communication between the nurse and the patient.

(2) Tactile communication between healthy and ill individuals can have highly beneficial results.

c. Therapeutic touch may make some patients uncomfortable; you are entering their personal space and their feelings must be respected, so make sure you ask the patient if he/she would like a back rub.

d. Agents used for back massage.

(1) Lotions or emollients.

(a) Lotions and emollients reduce friction and lubricate the skin.

(b) They are appropriate for most patients, especially those with a tendency toward dry skin; that is, elderly patients.

(2) Rubbing alcohol.

(a) Alcohol evaporates quickly, so it has a cooling but very drying effect.

(b) A certain amount of alcohol is absorbed by the skin so it should not be used on infants, elderly patients, or patients with liver disease.

(3) Powder.

(a) Powder reduces friction but also has a drying effect on the skin.

(b) It may be appropriate for those patients who perspire freely and/or are confined to bed.

e. General guidelines.

(1) A back massage should take about five to ten minutes and can be given with the patient's bath, before bedtime, or at any other time during the day.

(2) Determine if any patient allergies or skin sensitivities exist before applying lotion to the patient's skin.

(3) The greatest relaxation effect of a massage occurs when the rhythm of the massage is coordinated with the patient's breathing.

## 3-11. GUIDELINES FOR SHAVING A MALE PATIENT

a. If the patient is alert, question him about his shaving habits, and follow his routine as closely as possible.

(1) Gather equipment and supplies.

(a) Towels.

(b) Washcloth.

(c) Basin with hot water.

(d) Shaving cream.

(e) Razor.

(f) Soap.

(g) Aftershave lotion.

(2) Wet the wash cloth, wring out any excess moisture, and apply it to the beard area (to soften the beard).

(3) Apply shaving cream to the beard.

(4) Shave the beard on the cheeks and upper lip in the direction that the hair grows.

(5) Shave the beard on the neck against the direction of the hair growth.

(6) Wash off any remaining shaving cream.

(7) With clean water, finish washing the patient's face.

b. Always use an electric razor on patients with bleeding disorders to prevent uncontrollable bleeding from facial cuts.

c. Do not use plugged in electric razors on patients who are receiving oxygen therapy because of the danger of combustion; safety razors or rechargeable battery operated shavers are safe.

d. Consult with the charge nurse before shaving any patient who has had facial surgery or who may have hemophilia.

e. Patients who are combative, suicidal, or disoriented should have supervision and assistance while shaving.

## 3-12. PERINEAL CARE

a. Perineal care is often referred to as "pericare;" it consists of external irrigation of the vulva and perineum following voiding or defecation and is part of the routine A. M. and P. M. care.

b. Patients may be able to perform their own perineal care or may need partial or total assistance from the nurse.

c. Embarrassment on the part of the patient and the nurse can be effectively dealt with by ensuring patient privacy during the procedure and not totally exposing the patient's genital area.

d. Key points.

(1) Ensure patient privacy.

(2) Wipe from front to back (vagina toward rectum) on female patients to avoid contaminating the vagina or urethral meatus.

(3) Do not use the same washcloth for any other portion of the patient's bath.

## 3-13. BED PATIENT'S HAIR CARE

a. **Principles for Shampooing the Bed Patient's Hair**.

(1) The supine position is preferred for weaker patients.

(2) Patients with significant heart or lung disease will not tolerate being supine; they must be in a sitting position.

(3) Hair care should be given regularly during illness, just as it would be normally.

b. **Purposes of Hair Care**.

(1) Hair care improves the morale of the patient.

(2) It stimulates the circulation of the scalp.

c. Shampooing removes bacteria, microorganisms, oils, and dirt that cling to the hair.

## 3-14. CLOSING.

Nothing points out loss of independence quite as much as an inability to perform personal hygiene unassisted. Your thoughtfulness and the professionalism you exhibit when assisting a patient with hygiene needs will foster that patient's feelings of independence, confidence, trust, and comfort.

***Continue with Exercises***

## EXERCISES, LESSON 3

**INSTRUCTIONS.** The following exercises are to be answered by completing the incomplete statement or by writing the answer in the space provided at the end of the question.

After you have completed all the exercises, turn to "Solutions to Exercises" at the end of the lesson and check your answers.

1. Confinement in bed increases perspiration __________________ growth is stimulated by moisture.

2. Skin irritation from hospital bed linens may result in skin breakdown and subsequent ______________________.

3. Continuous pressure over any body part impairs circulation to that part and can cause skin breakdown and eventual ________________________.

4. If the patient is incontinent, skin breakdown is likely to occur due to the presence of moisture and ___________________ on the skin.

5. At the first sign of redness to the skin, the area should be washed with soap and water and rubbed with ___________________

6. If you notice signs of pressure on a patient's skin, report it to the _____________.

7. Patient hygiene procedures followed in the morning affect the patient's _________________ throughout the day; care received at the end of the day relaxes the patient and influences the ability to ________________

8. At the end of the day, it is important to check the floor for items such as ___________ and _______________, which the patient could slip on or fall over.

9. After a patient's bedside bath, be sure the ____________________ are up and the ____________________ is within reach.

10. Respect for the patient's ____________________ decreases the patient's emotional discomfort during personal care.

11. For a bedside bath, maintain bath water between ______ °F and _______ °F.

12. During the bathing procedure, observe any abnormal skin condition; describe the location, color, size, and how it __________ to the patient.

13. An abnormal body odor may be an indication of infection or _____________ disease.

14. Hot skin could mean fever; cold skin could mean ________________________.

15. Oral hygiene is especially important for patients who breath through their mouths, because their oral __________________ dries out quickly.

16. Name three types of observations made during oral care, which must be recorded.

    a. _________________________________.

    b. _________________________________.

    c. _________________________________.

17. Dentures must be kept in _______________ to preserve their fit and general quality.

18. When rinsing dentures, be careful NOT to use _______ water.

19. Mouthwash and other solutions that contain _______________ should not be used for the patient with ulcerations, as they are frequently very painful.

20. If the patient is unconscious, oral care should be performed every ____ hours.

21. Lotions and emollients used during a back massage reduce ____________ and lubricate the skin.

22. A certain amount of alcohol is absorbed by the skin during back massage; therefore, it should not be used on infants, elderly patients, or patients with _________ disease.

23. Always use an electric razor on patients with ________________ disorders.

24. When performing perineal care, it is important to remember to wipe from _____________ to ____________________________ on female patients.

25. The _______________ position is preferred during hair care for weaker patients.

26. Patient with significant heart or lung disease must be in a _____________ position during hair care.

***Check Your Answers on Next Page***

**SOLUTIONS TO EXERCISES, LESSON 3**

1. Bacterial. (para 3-2a(1))

2. Infection. (para 3-2a(2))

3. Ulcerations. (para 3-3a)

4. Bacteria. (para 3-3b)

5. Lotion. (para 3-4b)

6. Charge nurse. (para 3-4c)

7. Comfort, sleep. (para 3-5a(1) and b(1))

8. Chairs, linens. (para 3-5b(3))

9. Side rails, call light. (paras 3-6a(2), (3))

10. Privacy. (para 3-6b(1))

11. 110, 115. (para 3-6c(4))

12. Feels. (para 3-7a(2))

13. Kidney. (para 3-7a(3)(b))

14. Poor circulation. (para 3-7a(3)(e))

15. Mucosa. (para 3-8b(2))

16. A correct answer consists of any three of the following:

    Bleeding.
    Swelling of gums.
    Unusual mouth odor.
    Effect of brushing the teeth. (paras 3-8c(1)-(4))

17. Water. (para 3-8d(1)(d))

18. Hot. (para 3-8d(4))

19. Alcohol. (para 3-8e(3)(c))

20. Four. (para 3-8f(1))

21. Friction. (para 3-10d(1)(a))

22. Liver. (para 3-10d(2)(b))

23. Bleeding. (para 3-11b)

24. Front, back (vagina to rectum). (para 3-12d(2))

25. Supine. (para 3-13a(1))

26. Sitting. (para 3-13a(2))

***END OF LESSON 3***

## LESSON ASSIGNMENT

**LESSON 4** Body Mechanics.

**LESSON ASSIGNMENT** Paragraphs 4-1 through 4-21.

**LESSON OBJECTIVES** After completing this lesson, you should be able to:

4-1. Define and identify principles of good body mechanics.

4-2. Identify techniques of body mechanics used when performing work.

4-3. Name the eight general considerations for performing physical tasks.

4-4. Identify reasons for using good body mechanics.

4-5. Identify reasons for changing the position of a patient.

4-6. Identify basic principles for positioning and turning patients.

4-7. Identify techniques for maintaining proper body alignment of the patient lying on his/her back.

4-8. Identify descriptions of positions used when positioning a patient.

4-9. Identify steps used to adjust the backrest and pillows of a patient in a gatch bed.

4-10. Identify actions, which can be taken by a nurse to alleviate discomfort and promote relaxation of a patient.

4-11. Select rationales for getting a patient out of bed.

4-12. Identify principles for assisting patients out of bed.

4-13. Identify steps used in preparing to ambulate a patient and stages of ambulation.

4-14. Identify actions, which should be taken if a patient begins to fall.

**SUGGESTION**

After studying the assignment, complete the exercises at the end of this lesson. These exercises will help you to achieve the lesson objectives.

# LESSON 4

# BODY MECHANICS

## Section I. TECHNIQUES OF BODY MECHANICS

### 4-1. INTRODUCTION

Some of the most common injuries sustained by members of the health care team are severe musculoskeletal strains. Many injuries can be avoided by the conscious use of proper body mechanics when performing physical labor.

### 4-2. DEFINITION

Body mechanics is the utilization of correct muscles to complete a task safely and efficiently, without undue strain on any muscle or joint.

### 4-3. PRINCIPLES OF GOOD BODY MECHANICS

a. **Maintain a Stable Center of Gravity**.

(1) Keep your center of gravity low.

(2) Keep your back straight.

(3) Bend at the knees and hips.

b. **Maintain a Wide Base of Support**. This will provide you with maximum stability while lifting.

(1) Keep your feet apart.

(2) Place one foot slightly ahead of the other.

(3) Flex your knees to absorb jolts.

(4) Turn with your feet.

c. **Maintain the Line of Gravity**. The line should pass vertically through the base of support.

(1) Keep your back straight.

(2) Keep the object being lifted close to your body.

d. **Maintain Proper Body Alignment**.

(1) Tuck in your buttocks.

(2) Pull your abdomen in and up.

(3) Keep your back flat.

(4) Keep your head up.

(5) Keep your chin in.

(6) Keep your weight forward and supported on the outside of your feet.

## 4-4. TECHNIQUES OF BODY MECHANICS

a. **Lifting.**

(1) Use the stronger leg muscles for lifting.

(2) Bend at the knees and hips; keep your back straight.

(3) Lift straight upward, in one smooth motion.

b. **Reaching**.

(1) Stand directly in front of and close to the object.

(2) Avoid twisting or stretching.

(3) Use a stool or ladder for high objects.

(4) Maintain a good balance and a firm base of support.

(5) Before moving the object, be sure that it is not too large or too heavy.

c. **Pivoting**.

(1) Place one foot slightly ahead of the other.

(2) Turn both feet at the same time, pivoting on the heel of one foot and the toe of the other.

(3) Maintain a good center of gravity while holding or carrying the object.

d. **Avoid Stooping**.

(1) Squat (bending at the hips and knees).

(2) Avoid stooping (bending at the waist).

(3) Use your leg muscles to return to an upright position.

## 4-5. GENERAL CONSIDERATIONS FOR PERFORMING PHYSICAL TASKS

a. It is easier to pull, push, or roll an object than it is to lift it.

b. Movements should be smooth and coordinated rather than jerky.

c. Less energy or force is required to keep an object moving than it is to start and stop it.

d. Use the arm and leg muscles as much as possible, the back muscles as little as possible.

e. Keep the work as close as possible to your body. It puts less of a strain on your back, legs, and arms.

f. Rock backward or forward on your feet to use your body weight as a pushing or pulling force.

g. Keep the work at a comfortable height to avoid excessive bending at the waist.

h. Keep your body in good physical condition to reduce the chance of injury.

## 4-6. REASONS FOR THE USE OF PROPER BODY MECHANICS

Use proper body mechanics in order to avoid the following:

a. Excessive fatigue.

b. Muscle strains or tears.

c. Skeletal injuries.

d. Injury to the patient.

e. Injury to assisting staff members.

## 4-7. STEPS INVOLVED IN PROPERLY MOVING AN OBJECT TO A NEW LOCATION

The following paragraph takes you through the process of moving (lifting, pivoting, squatting, and carrying) a heavy object. (The same rules would apply to moving a patient.) The object will be moved from a waist high area to a lower area five to ten feet away. The procedure will combine all the rules of body mechanics previously discussed.

a. Identify the object to be moved.

b. Adopt a stable base of support.

(1) Your feet are separated.

(2) One foot is behind the other.

(3) Your back is straight.

c. Grasp the object at its approximate center of gravity.

d. Pull the object toward your body's center of gravity using your arm and leg muscles.

e. Re-establish your base of support and appropriate body alignment.

(1) Your back is straight.

(2) You have a stable base of support.

(3) You are holding the object approximately at waist height and close to your body.

f. Pivot toward the desired direction of travel.

(1) Turn on both feet at the same time.

(2) Maintain a stable balance.

g. Re-establish a stable base of support and appropriate body alignment.

(1) Your back is straight.

(2) Your feet are apart, one slightly behind the other.

(3) The object is at hip level, close to your body.

h. Squat and place the object onto the lower area.

(1) Bend at the knees and hips.

(2) Maintain a straight back.

(3) Maintain a stable base of support.

(4) Use your arm and leg muscles (as needed) for guidance.

(5) Use your leg muscles to resume an upright position.

## Section II. POSITIONING AND AMBULATING THE ADULT PATIENT

### 4-8. INTRODUCTION

One of the basic procedures that nursing personnel perform most frequently is that of changing the patient's position. Any position, even the most comfortable one, will become unbearable after a period of time. Whereas the healthy person has the ability to move at will, the sick person's movements may be limited by disease, injury, or helplessness. It is often the responsibility of the practical nurse to position the patient and change his position frequently. Once the patient is able to ambulate, certain precautions must be taken to ensure the patient's safety.

### 4-9. REASONS FOR CHANGING THE POSITION OF A PATIENT

The following are reasons for changing a patient's position.

a. To promote comfort and relaxation.

b. To restore body function.

(1) Changing positions improves gastrointestinal function.

(2) It also improves respiratory function.

(a) Changing positions allows for greater lung expansion.

(b) It relieves pressure on the diaphragm.

c. To prevent deformities.

(1) When one lies in bed for long periods of time, muscles become atonic and atrophy.

(2) Prevention of deformities will allow the patient to ambulate when his activity level is advanced.

d. To relieve pressure and prevent strain (which lead to the formation of decubiti).

e. To stimulate circulation.

f. To give treatments (that is), range of motion exercises).

## 4-10. BASIC PRINCIPLES IN POSITIONING OF PATIENTS

a. Maintain good patient body alignment. Think of the patient in bed as though he were standing.

b. Maintain the patient's safety.

c. Reassure the patient to promote comfort and cooperation.

d. Properly handle the patient's body to prevent pain or injury.

e. Keep in mind proper body mechanics for the practical nurse.

f. Obtain assistance, if needed, to move heavy or helpless patients.

g. Follow specific physician's orders.

h. A physician's order, such as one of the following, is needed for the patient to be out of bed.

(1) "Up ad lib."

(2) "Up as desired."

(3) "OOB" (out of bed).

i. Do not use special devices (that is., splints, traction) unless ordered. Ask if you do not know what is allowed.

## 4-11. TURNING THE ADULT PATIENT

a. **General Principles for Turning the Adult Patient**.

(1) Sometimes the physician will specify how often to turn a patient.

(a) A schedule can be set up for turning the adult patient throughout his "awake" hours.

(b) The patient should be rotated through four positions (unless a particular position is contraindicated):

1 Prone (see figure 4-1 and paragraph 4-13c).

2 Supine (figure 4-2 and paragraph 4-13a).

3 Left Sim's (figure 4-3).

4 Right Sim's (figure 4-3).

(c) Plan a schedule and follow it.

(d) Record the position change each time to ensure that all positions are used.

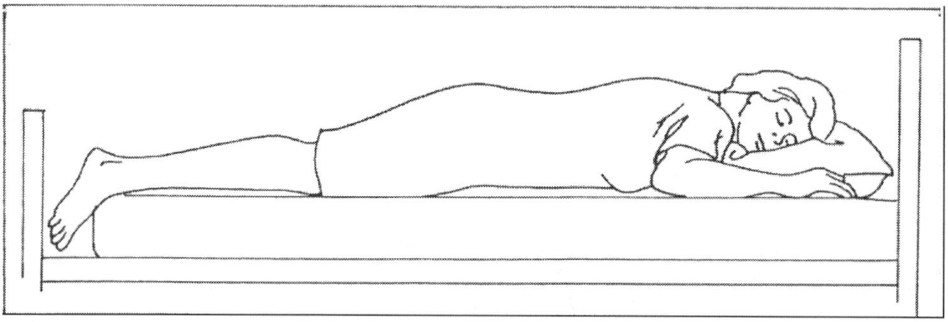

Figure 4-1. Prone position.

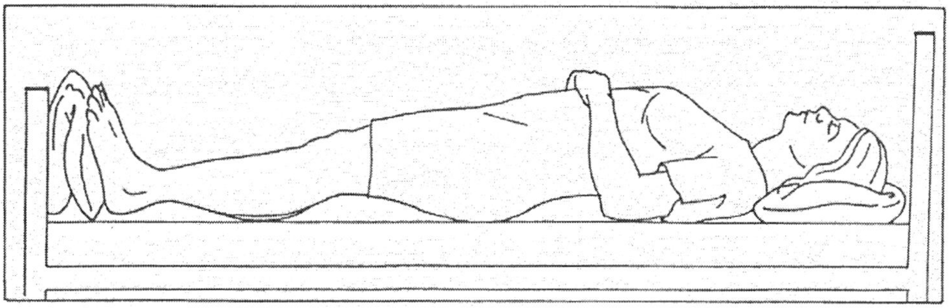

Figure 4-2. Supine position.

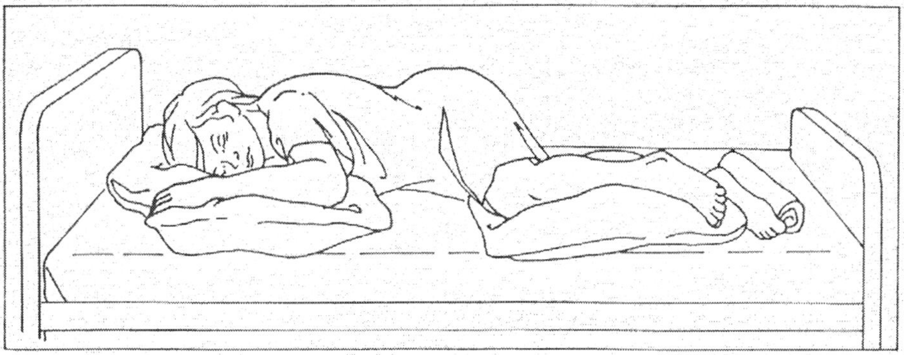

Figure 4-3. Sim's position.

(e) One example of a schedule for turning would be:

1000--Prone position
1200--Left Sim's position
1400--Supine position
1600--Right Sim's position
1800--Prone position

1 Notice that in the preceding sequence, the patient is required to make only a quarter turn rather than a half turn each time the position is changed.

2 If the patient experiences pain while turning, a quarter turn will be less painful than a half turn.

(2) Certain conditions may make it impossible to turn the patient.

(a) Turning may be impossible if the patient has fractures that require traction appliances.

(b) Turning may be harmful to patients with spinal injuries.

(c) In these cases, you need to rub the back by lifting the patient slightly off the bed and massaging with your hand held flat.

(d) It is especially important to prevent skin breakdowns in the person who lies on his back for long periods of time.

**NOTE**: For the initial development of skin breakdown, a patient does not have to lie on his back for long periods of time, especially if moisture and sheet wrinkles are present.

(e) You may want to turn a patient only to wash or rub the back or change the bed.

b. **Logrolling** (see figure 4-4).

(1) Description.

(a) Logrolling is a technique used to turn a patient whose body must at all times be kept in a straight alignment (like a log).

(b) This technique is used for the patient who has a spinal injury.

(c) Logrolling is used for the patient who must be turned in one movement, without twisting.

(d) Logrolling requires two people, or if the patient is large, three people.

(2) Technique.

(a) Wash your hands.

(b) Approach and identify the patient (by checking the identification band) and explain the procedure (using simple terms and pointing out the benefits).

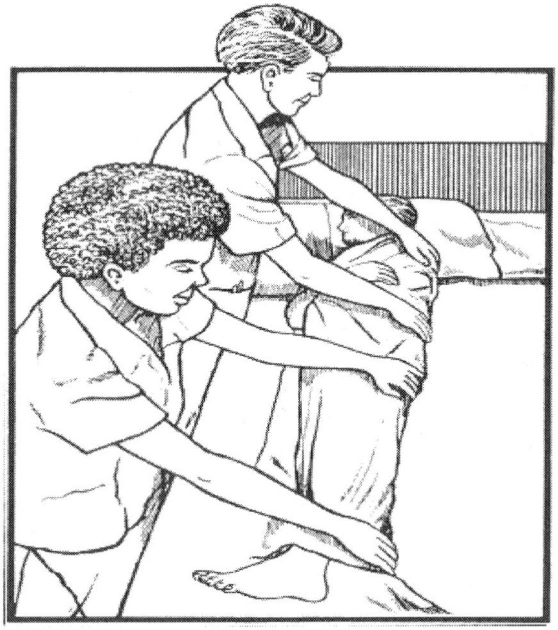

Figure 4-4. Logrolling.

(c) Provide privacy.

(d) Position the bed.

1 The bed should be in the flat position at a comfortable working height.

2 Lower the side rail on the side of the body at which you are working.

(e) Position yourself with your feet apart and your knees flexed close to the side of the bed.

(f) Fold the patient's arms across his chest.

(g) Place your arms under the patient so that a major portion of the patient's weight is centered between your arms. The arm of one nurse should support the patient's head and neck.

(h) On the count of three, move the patient to the side of the bed, rocking backward on your heels and keeping the patient's body in correct alignment.

(i) Raise the side rail on that side of the bed.

(j) Move to the other side of the bed.

(k) Place a pillow under the patient's head and another between his legs.

(l) Position the patient's near arm toward you.

(m) Grasp the far side of the patient's body with your hands evenly distributed from the shoulder to the thigh.

(n) On the count of three, roll the patient to a lateral position, rocking backward onto your heels.

(o) Place pillows in front of and behind the patient's trunk to support his alignment in the lateral position.

(p) Provide for the patient's comfort and safety.

1 Position the call bell.

2 Place personal items within reach.

3 Be sure the side rails are up and secure.

(q) Report and record as appropriate.

**4-12. MAINTAINING PROPER BODY ALIGNMENT WITH THE PATIENT ON HIS BACK**

a. Patients who must lie on their backs much of the time should be kept as comfortable as possible to prevent body deformities. The paraplegic and quadriplegic may not be able to tell you if their position is uncomfortable. You must be especially attentive in this case to prevent possible problems from malalignment.

b. Pillows can be used to support the patient's head, neck, arms, and hands and a footboard used to support the feet.

(1) Proper alignment gives respiratory and digestive organs room to function normally.

(2) The footboard is slanted to support the feet at right angles to the leg (a normal angle) and prevent foot drop.

c. If the patient's trunk must lie flatter than the neck and head:

(1) The patient should have only one pillow to support the head and neck.

(2) The patient may have a pillow placed under the legs to prevent pressure on the heels.

## 4-13. COMMON POSITIONS UTILIZED FOR THE ADULT PATIENT

a. **Placing the Adult Patient in the Supine Position** (see figure 4-2).

(1) Collect equipment.

(a) Pillows.

(b) Positioning aids as indicated.

(2) Wash your hands.

(3) Approach and identify the patient (by checking the identification band) and explain the procedure (using simple terms and pointing out the benefits).

(4) Provide privacy throughout the procedure.

(5) Position the bed.

(a) Place the bed in a flat or level position at working height, unless contraindicated.

(b) Lower the side rails on the proximal side (as necessary).

(6) Move the patient from a lateral (side) position to a supine position.

(a) For the patient on his side, remove supportive pillows.

(b) Fold top bedding back to the hips, being careful to avoid any undue exposure of the patient's body.

(c) With one hand on the patient's shoulder and one on the hip, roll his body in one piece (like a log) over onto his back.

(7) Align the patient's body in good position.

(a) Head, neck, and spine are in a straight line.

(b) Arms are at the patient's sides (parallel to the body) with hands prone.

(c) Legs are parallel to his body.

(d) Hips, knees, and feet should be in good alignment.

(8) Support the body parts in good alignment for comfort.

(a) Place a pillow under the head and shoulders to prevent strain on neck muscles and hyperextension and flexion of the neck.

(b) Support the small of the back with a folded bath towel or small pillow.

(c) Put a footboard at the foot of the bed and place the feet flat against it (at right angles to the legs) to prevent plantar flexion ("foot drop").

(d) Arrange a sandbag along the outer portion of the right foot to keep the foot upright.

(e) Make a trochanter roll and arrange it along the right hip and thigh to keep the hip joint from rotating outward.

(f) Place a pillow under each forearm so the arm is at least six inches from the body.

(9) Provide for the patient's comfort and safety.

(a) Replace the bedding neatly and raise the side rails, if used.

(b) Place the call light within reach.

(c) Position the bedside stand or overbed table so that the patient will be within easy reach of drinking water and personal items.

(d) Leave the bed in the low position.

(10) Report significant nursing observations to the charge nurse.

b. **Placing the Adult Patient in the Fowler's and Semi-Fowler's Position** (see figures 4-5 and 4-6).

(1) Collect equipment.

(a) Pillows.

(b) Positioning aids as indicated.

(2) Wash your hands.

(3) Approach and identify the patient (checking the ID band) and explain the procedure (in simple terms and pointing out benefits).

(4) Provide for privacy throughout the procedure.

(5) Be sure the patient is in a supine position with his head near the top of the bed.

(6) Elevate the head of the bed.

(a) Elevate 60 to 90 degrees for the Fowler's position.

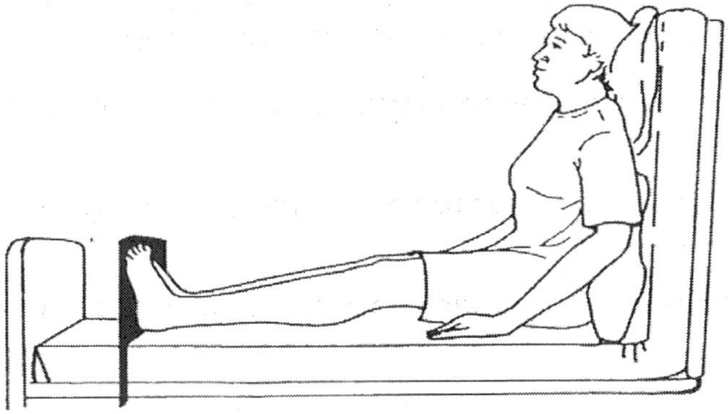

Figure 4-5. Fowler's position.

(b) Elevate 45 to 60 degrees for the semi-Fowler's position.

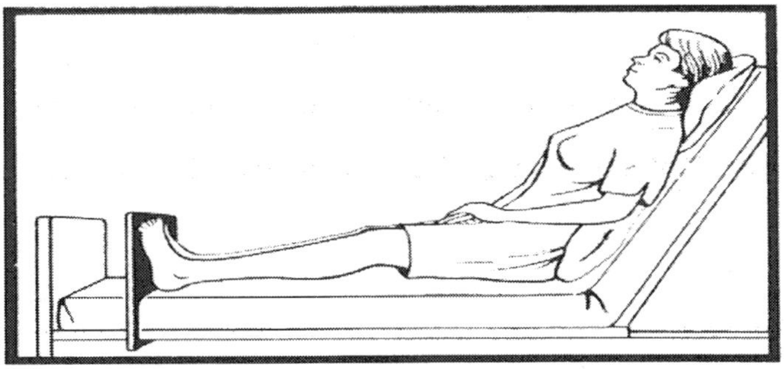

Figure 4-6. Semi-Fowler's position.

(7) Raise the knee gatch (knee rest) of the bed approximately 15 degrees unless contraindicated.

(8) Use a footboard to maintain the feet at right angles to the legs.

(9) Use pillows for support as needed.

(a) Behind the shoulders and head to prevent flexion and hyperextension of the neck.

(b) Behind the lower back to prevent posterior convexity of the lumbar spine region.

(c) Under the thighs to prevent hyperextension of the knees.

(10) Place the patient in good body alignment.

(a) Head, neck, and back are straight.

(b) The weight of the body is supported where the hips are flexed in the sitting position.

(c) Feet are straight.

(d) Toes are pointing up.

(11) Provide for the patient's comfort and safety.

(a) Replace bedding neatly.

(b) Raise and secure the side rails.

(c) Place the call light within reach.

(d) Position the bedside stand or overbed table so that the patient will be within easy reach of drinking water and personal items.

(e) Leave the bed in a low position.

(12) Report significant nursing observations to the charge nurse.

c. **Prone Position** (see figure 4-1).

(1) Collect the equipment.

(a) Pillows.

(b) Positioning aids as indicated.

(2) Wash your hands.

(3) Approach and identify the patient and explain the procedure.

(4) Provide for privacy.

(5) Adjust the bed.

(a) Lower the headrest and knee rest so that the bed is in a flat position.

(b) Raise the bed to working height.

(c) Lower the side rails on the side where you are working.

(d) Fold the top bedding down to the level of the patient's hips, but avoid undue exposure of the patient's body, which may cause embarrassment.

(6) Position the patient in bed.

(a) If there is room between the end of the mattress and the foot of the bed, the patient should be moved down in the bed so that his feet extend over the edge of the mattress.

(b) Remove the footboard if one is present.

(7) Turn the patient onto his side and then onto his stomach.

(a) Roll toward you so you can observe him closely.

(b) Continue to roll until he is on his stomach.

(8) Align the patient in good position.

(a) Head is turned to one side.

(b) Neck and back are in a straight line.

(c) Arms are parallel to the body in a slightly flexed position; or arm on the same side toward which the head is turned can be flexed sharply at the elbow so the hand is near the head.

1 Legs are straight.

2 Feet are extended over the edge of the mattress to avoid hyperextension of the foot; or a pillow is placed under both ankles to prevent plantar flexion (foot drop) as a result of prolonged hyperextension.

(d) Support the patient's body and keep it in good alignment.

1 A small pillow or folded towel under the head may be used to prevent hyperextension and flexion of the neck.

2 A pillow under the abdomen provides comfort and prevents hyperextension of the lower spine.

(e) Provide for the patient's comfort and safety.

1 Replace bedding neatly.

2 Raise and secure the side rails.

3 Place the call light within reach.

4 Position the bedside stand or over-the-bed table within reach so the patient can get drinking water and personal items.

5 Leave the bed in a low position.

(f) Report significant nursing observations to the Charge Nurse.

d. **Lateral** (see figure 4-7) **and Sim's** (see figure 4-3) **Positions.**

(1) Collect equipment.

(a) Pillows.

(b) Positioning aids as indicated.

(2) Wash hands.

(3) Approach and identify the patient by checking identification band.

(4) Explain the procedure and gain patient's cooperation.

(a) Use simple terms.

(b) Point out benefits.

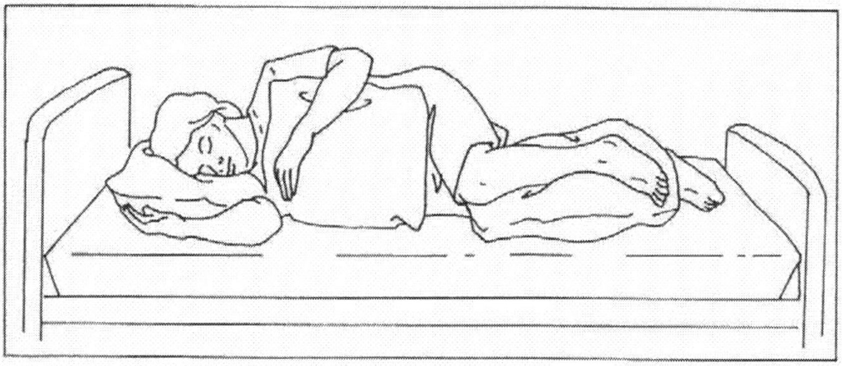

Figure 4-7. Lateral position.

(5) Provide for privacy.

(6) Position the bed.

(a) Lower head and foot of the bed so it is level or flat.

(b) Lower the side rails on the proximal side; the distal side rail must be up.

(7) Turn the patient onto the side.

(a) Obtain assistance, if needed.

(b) Fold the top bedding back to the level of the patient's hips, but avoid undue exposure of the patient's body which may cause embarrassment.

(c) Flex the distal knee and place the distal arm across the chest.

(d) "Log-roll" the patient toward you by placing one hand on the shoulder and the other on the distal hip and pulling without twisting the patient's torso.

(e) Reach behind the patient's back with both hands, placing one on the proximal hip and lift slightly outward and roll the body toward yourself.

(8) Alternative method: turn the patient onto the side away from self.

(a) "Log-roll" the patient's body away from self by putting one hand on the proximal shoulder and the other on the hip and rolling the patient to the distal side.

(b) Lower hands to the distal shoulder and hip and pull them toward self to stabilize the patient in the lateral position.

(9) Align the patient's body in good position.

(a) Ensure the patient is not lying on his/her arm.

(b) Head, neck, and back are in a straight line.

(c) Legs are parallel with knees slightly flexed.

(d) Uppermost arm may be flexed across patient's abdomen or supported on his/her body and hip.

(10) Support the body in good alignment for comfort.

(a) Place a pillow under the patient's head and neck to prevent muscle strain and maintain alignment.

(b) Put a pillow under the uppermost leg so that it is supported from the knee to the foot.

(c) Place another pillow firmly against the patient's abdomen to support the back and hips in better alignment, if necessary.

(d) You may want to use a pillow to support the back.

1 Place a pillow lengthwise along the back.

2 Tuck one edge under the side.

3 Roll the remainder of the pillow under (toward the bed surface).

4 Tuck the pillow firmly against the back.

(e) You may also want to use a pillow to support the knee.

1 Place a pillow between the knees.

2 Bend the upper knee to provide stability.

(11) Provide for the patient's comfort and safety.

(a) Replace the bedding neatly.

(b) Raise and secure the side rails.

(c) Place the call light within reach.

(d) Position the bedside stand and over-the-bed table so that the patient is within easy reach of drinking water and personal items.

(e) Leave the bed in a low position.

(12) Report significant nursing observations to the charge nurse.

## 4-14. ACTIONS THE PRACTICAL NURSE CAN TAKE TO ALLEVIATE DISCOMFORT AND PROMOTE RELAXATION

a. Obtain comfortable bedding. Allow some of patient's own possessions (such as a pillow or afghan) when possible.

b. Change the bed position (head and knee).

c. Reduce the noise and light in the patient's room.

d. Check for mechanical reasons for discomfort:

(1) Bed linens or Chux® which are gathered and wrinkled under the patient.

(2) Plastic mattress covers that wrinkle and cause pressure.

(3) Top covers which may be pulled too tightly over the feet and legs.

(4) The patient lying on tubes, drains, syringe caps, or other equipment.

(5) Soiled dressings, urine, and feces causing the bed to be wet.

(6) Nonfunctioning equipment, to include alarms sounding without cause.

## 4-15. POSITIONING THE ADULT TO PROMOTE SLEEP AND RELAXATION

If a patient is restless, having difficulty getting comfortable, or not sleeping well, consider the following steps. As always, be sure you have a physician's order for the patient to be turned when necessary.

a. Wash your hands.

b. Approach and identify the patient (by checking the ID band) and explain the procedure (using simple terms and pointing out the benefits).

c. Perform practical nursing care to promote relaxation.

(1) Straighten or change the linens.

(2) Give the patient a back massage.

(3) Provide oral hygiene.

(4) Administer hair care.

(5) Administer a sponge bath and get fresh pajamas.

d. Position the patient in the preferred position for rest if possible. Follow the physician's order for turning if specified.

e. Modify the position for support and comfort. Use aids for the patient's positioning as indicated.

f. Check for the position and function of tubes and drains.

g. Check the bed linens for comfort.

(1) Wrinkles in linens.

(2) Wrinkles in mattress cover.

(3) Tightness over the feet and lower extremities.

h. Tell the patient when you plan to return.

i. Position the call light and bedside table within easy reach.

**NOTE:** To keep the call light within the patient's reach, secure it to the bed linen with a safety pin, if necessary.

j. Provide for quiet in the area when possible.

(1) Close the doors.

(2) Turn off any radios or TVs.

(3) Ask unnecessary visitors and personnel to leave the area.

k. Avoid interrupting the patient once he falls asleep.

(1) Schedule medications for times when the patient is being turned.

(2) Keep nursing care treatments and procedures to a minimum during sleep hours.

l. Report and record significant nursing observations.

## 4-16. RATIONALE FOR GETTING THE PATIENT OUT OF BED

a. Preserve or improve muscle tone.

b. Improve circulation, particularly in the lower extremities.

c. Preserve pulmonary tissue and airway function.

d. Preserve muscle and joint mobility.

## 4-17. PRINCIPLES OF ASSISTING PATIENTS OUT OF BED

a. Reassure the patient of his personal safety against injury and over-exertion.

b. If necessary, get additional help to assist you in ambulating the patient.

c. Support the affected side or extremities of the patient when ambulating or moving.

d. Do not overtire the patient; increase time up in the chair and ambulation gradually.

e. Lock all wheelchair or litter wheels before transferring the patient from the bed.

f. Stabilize the footstool, when it is utilized.

g. Place a signal cord or call-light button within easy reach of the patient while he is up.

h. Check on the patient frequently.

## 4-18. STEPS IN PREPARING TO AMBULATE THE PATIENT

a. Review the patient's medical record for an authorizing physician's order.

b. Review the patient's nursing care plan for information regarding the following:

(1) Physical limitations.

(2) Mechanical equipment being utilized; that is, IV infusion pumps, chest drainage set, urinary drainage sets.

(3) Distance patient is to ambulate.

(4) Length of time patient is to be out of bed.

(5) Frequency patient is to get out of bed.

c. Review the Nurse's Notes to identify the patient's previous tolerance of the activity specified.

d. Explain the rationale for getting out of bed to the patient.

e. Pre-medicate for pain prior to getting out of bed, if necessary.

f. Ensure that the patient is appropriately clothed, including footwear.

## 4-19. STAGES IN ASSISTING THE PATIENT TO AMBULATE

a. Assist the patient to sit on the side of the bed (dangling).

b. Assist the patient to stand.

c. Assist the patient to move to a chair, or to ambulate.

## 4-20. MANAGEMENT OF THE FALLING PATIENT

a. **The Patient Who Collapses**.

(1) Assume a broad stance with one foot slightly forward, grasp the patient's body firmly at the waist or under the axilla, and allow him to slide down against your leg.

(2) Ease the patient slowly to the floor using your body as an incline.

(3) Lower your body along with the patient, if necessary.

(4) Utilize proper body mechanics.

b. **The Patient Who Loses Balance**.

(1) Attempt to stabilize the patient by bracing him against you.

(2) Guide the patient to the bedside or chair, if possible.

(3) If a fall begins to occur, guide him slowly toward the floor.

## 4-21. CLOSING

The physiological and psychological benefits of repositioning, being out of bed, and sitting up or ambulating should not be under-emphasized. Basic nursing care activity such as this, although not always pleasant for the patient, does make a significant difference in the recovery and return to health of the patient.

*Continue with Exercises*

*Return to Table of Contents*

**EXERCISES, LESSON 4**

**INSTRUCTION:** Answer the following exercises by marking the lettered response that provides the best answer, by completing the statement, or by writing your response in the space provided in the exercise.

After you have completed the exercises, turn to the "Solution to Exercises" at the end of this lesson and check your answers. For each exercise answered incorrectly, reread the material referenced with the solution.

1. Body mechanics is the use of correct muscles to complete a task safely and efficiently, without undue strain on any ______________or _________________

2. Good body mechanics requires that you keep your back ______________and bend at the __________ and _________

3. When lifting, keep your feet _________with one foot slightly ahead of the other _________ your knees to absorb jolts; turn with your _____________.

4. When reaching for an object, you should stand directly in front of and ______________ the object.

5. When performing physical tasks, use your ________ and ________ muscles as much as possible and your muscles as little as possible.

6. Name four problems you can avoid by using good body mechanics.

   a. _______________________________.

   b. _______________________________.

   c. _______________________________.

   d. _______________________________.

7. Changing a patient's position allows for greater _________ expansion and relieves pressure on the ___________________.

8. When a patient lies in bed for long periods of time, his muscles tend to become atonic and ____________________.

9. When positioning a patient, obtain assistance to move a heavy or

_______________ patient.

10. Unless being turned or a particular position is contraindicated, a patient should be rotated through which four positions?

    a. ______________________________.

    b. ______________________________.

    c. ______________________________.

    d. ______________________________.

11. What should be done to prevent pressure and strain if a patient has a spinal injury and cannot be turned?

    ____________________________________________________________

12. If you must turn a patient with a spinal injury, which method should you use?

    ________________.

13. Proper body alignment of a patient who must lie on his back for a long period of time gives ___________________and ____________________organs room to function normally.

14.Name the positions illustrated below:

a.____________________________

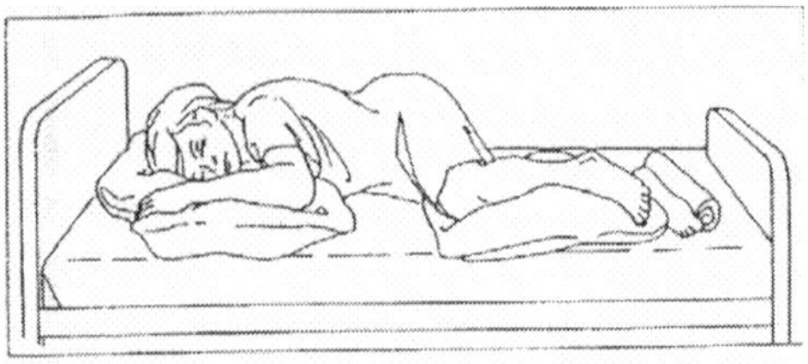

b. _________________________.

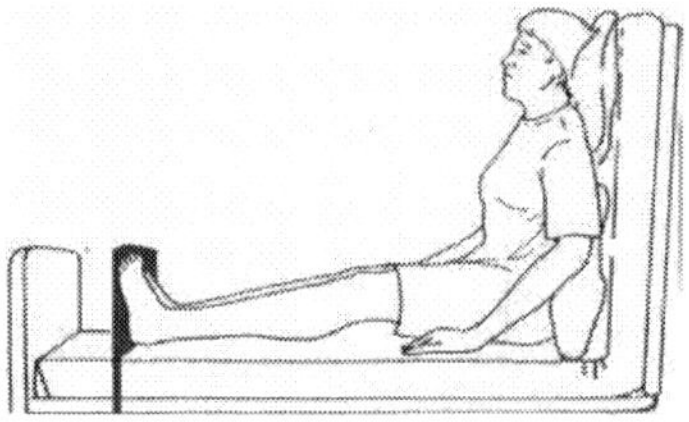

c. _________________________.

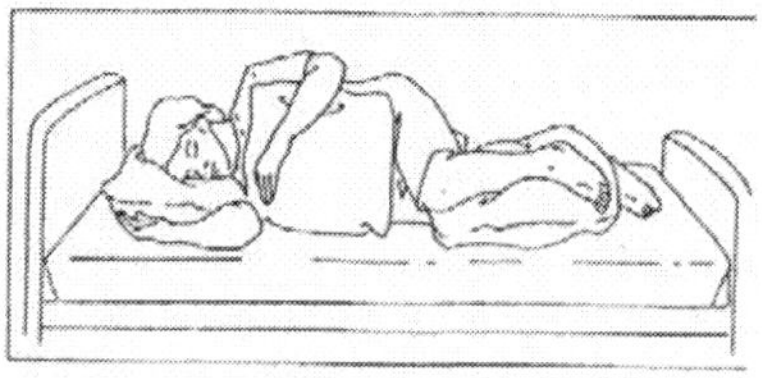

d. ____________________________.

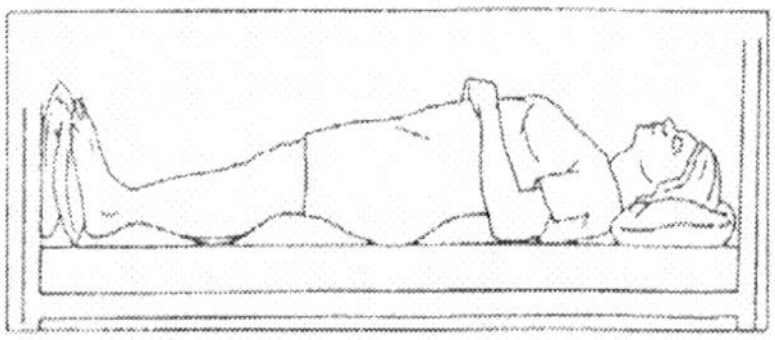

e. _________________________.

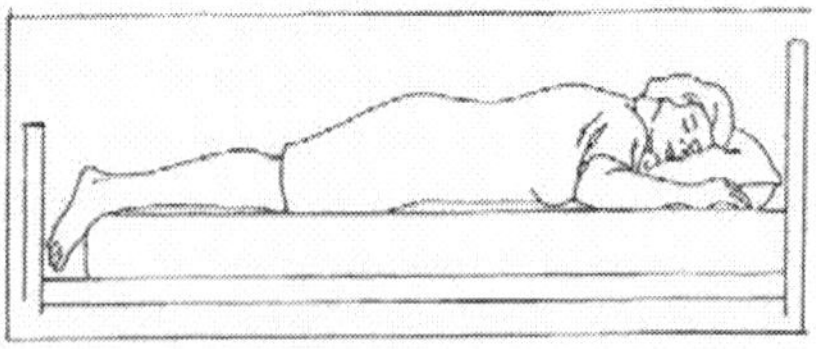

15. When placing an adult patient in the supine position, place a pillow under the head and shoulders to prevent strain on neck muscles and ____________________ and ____________________ of the neck.

16. Elevate the head of the bed _______ to _______ degrees for a patient in the Fowler's position and _______ to_______ degrees for Semi-Fowler's.

17. For a patient in the Fowler's or semi-Fowler's position, raise the knee gatch approximately ____degrees, unless contraindicated.

18. You are having difficulty keeping the call light within a patient's reach; what should you do?

    ______________________________________________________.

19. Name two things you can do to avoid interrupting a patient once he falls asleep.

    a. ______________________________.

    b. ______________________________.

20. Getting a patient out of bed improves his circulation, particularly in the ______________________.

21. Be sure to ______________________ all wheelchair or litter wheels before transferring a patient from the bed.

22. Before ambulating a patient, if necessary ____________________ for pain.

23. When managing a patient who has collapsed, assume a broad stance with one foot slightly ______________, grasp the patient's body firmly at the __________ or under the ______________, and allow him to slide down against your _______.

24. When managing a patient who has lost his balance, attempt to stabilize the patient by ____________________ against_____. Guide the patient to the __________ or __________ if possible.

25. When preparing to ambulate a patient, you should review the patient's _____________________, the patient's ______________________________, and the _______________________________________ .

*Check Your Answers on Next Page*

## SOLUTIONS TO EXERCISES, LESSON 4

1. Muscle, joint. (para 4-2)

2. Straight, knees, hips. (paras 4-3a(2), (3))

3. Apart, flex, feet. (paras 4-3b(1) -- (4))

4. Close to. (para 4-4b(1))

5. Arm, leg, back. (para 4-5d)

6. A correct answer consists of any four of the following:

   Excessive fatigue.
   Muscle strains or tears..
   Skeletal injuries.
   Injury to the patient.
   Injury to assisting staff members. (paras 4-6a--e)

7. Lung, diaphragm. (paras 4-9b(2)(a), (b))

8. Atrophy. (para 4-9c(1))

9. Helpless. (para 4-10f)

10. Prone, supine, left Sim's, right Sim's. (paras 4-11a(1)(b) 1 -- 4)

11. Rub the back by lifting the patient slightly off the bed and massaging with your hand held flat. (para 4-11a(2)(c))

12. Logrolling. (para 4-11b(1)(b))

13. Respiratory, digestive. (para 4-12b(1))

14. a. Sim's. (figure 4-3)
    b. Fowler's. (figure 4-5)
    c. Lateral. (figure 4-7)
    d. Supine. (figure 4-2)
    e. Prone. (figure 4-1)

15. Hyperextension, flexion. (para 4-13a(8)(a))

16. 60, 90, 45, 60. (paras 4-13b(6)(a), (b))

17. 15. (para 4-13b(7))

18. Secure it to the bed linen with a safety pin. (para 4-15i)

19. Schedule medications for times when the patient is being turned
Keep nursing care treatments and procedures to a minimum during sleep hours
(paras 4-15k(1), (2))

20. Lower extremities. (para 4-16b)

21. Lock. (para 4-17e

22. Pre-medicate. (para 4-18e)

23. Forward, waist, axilla, leg. (para 4-20a(1))

24. Bracing him, you, bedside, chair. (paras 4-20b(1), (2))

25. Medical record, nursing care plan, Nurse's Notes. (paras 4-18a, b, c)

***Return to Table of Contents***

## LESSON ASSIGNMENT

**LESSON 5** Active and Passive Range of Motion Exercises.

**TEXT ASSIGNMENT** Paragraphs 5-1 through 5-9.

**LESSON OBJECTIVES** After completing this lesson, you should be able to:

5-1. Identify the effects of immobility.

5-2. Identify the purposes of exercise for the immobile patient.

5-3. Define the five types of exercises.

5-4. Define the nine types of body movement.

5-5. Identify guidelines for range-of-motion exercises.

**SUGGESTION** After studying the assignment, complete the exercises at the end of this lesson. These exercises will help you to achieve the lesson objectives.

## LESSON 5

## ACTIVE AND PASSIVE RANGE OF MOTION EXERCISES

### 5-1. INTRODUCTION

The body was designed for motion. Regular exercise contributes to a healthy body; therefore immobility has a negative effect. A joint that has not been moved sufficiently can begin to stiffen within 24 hours and will eventually become inflexible. With longer periods of joint immobility, the tendons and muscles can be affected as well. Most people move and exercise their joints through the normal activities of daily living. When any joint cannot be moved in this way, the patient or nurse must move it at regular intervals to maintain muscle tone and joint mobility. Range of motion (ROM) exercises are ones in which a nurse or patient move each joint through as full a range as is possible without causing pain. The effect of both regular exercise and immobility on major body systems are discussed in this lesson.

### 5-2. THE EFFECTS OF IMMOBILITY

a. **Cardiovascular System.**

(1) Venous stasis caused by prolonged inactivity that restricts or slows venous circulation. Muscular activity, especially in the legs, helps move blood toward the central circulatory system.

(2) Increased cardiac workload due to increased viscosity from dehydration and decreased venous return. The heart works more when the body is resting, probably because there is less resistance offered by the blood vessels and because there is a change in the distribution of blood in the immobile person. The result is that the heart rate, cardiac output, and stroke volume increase.

(3) Thrombus and embolus formation caused by slow flowing blood, which may begin clotting within hours, and an increased rate in the coagulation of blood. During periods of immobility, calcium leaves bones and enters the blood, where it has an influence on blood coagulation.

(4) Orthostatic hypotension probably due to a decrease in the neurovascular reflexes, which normally causes vasoconstriction, and to a loss of muscle tone. The result is that blood pools and does not squeeze from veins in the lower part of the body to the central circulatory system. The immobile person is more susceptible to developing orthostatic hypotension. The person tends to feel weak and faint when the condition occurs.

b. **Respiratory System.**

(1) Hypostatic pneumonia. The depth and rate of respirations and the movement of secretions in the respiratory tract is decreased when a person is immobile. The pooling secretions and congestion predispose to respiratory tract infections. Signs and symptoms include:

(a) Increased temperature.

(b) Thick copious secretions.

(c) Cough.

(d) Increased pulse.

(e) Confusion, irritability, or disorientation.

(f) Sharp chest pain.

(g) Dyspnea.

(2) Atelectasis. When areas of lung tissue are not used over a period of time, incomplete expansion or collapse of lung tissue may occur.

(3) Impaired coughing. Impairment of coughing mechanism may be due to the patient's position in bed decreasing chest cage expansion.

c. **Musculoskeletal System**.

(1) Muscle atrophy. Disuse leads to decreased muscle size, tone, and strength.

(2) Contracture. Decreased joint movement leads to permanent shortening of muscle tissue, resistant to stretching. The strong flexor muscles pull tight, causing a contraction of the extremity or a permanent position of flexion.

(3) Ankylosis. Consolidation and immobility of a joint in a particular position due to contracture.

(4) Osteoporosis. Lack of stress on the bone causes an increase in calcium absorption, weakening the bone.

d. **Nervous System**.

(1) Altered sensation caused by prolonged pressure and continual stimulation of nerves. Usually pain is felt at first and then sensation is altered, and the patient no longer senses the pain.

(2) Peripheral nerve palsy.

e. **Gastrointestinal System.**

(1) Disturbance in appetite caused by the slowing of gastrointestinal tract, secondary immobility, and decreased activity resulting in anorexia.

(2) Altered digestion and utilization of nutrients resulting in constipation.

(3) Altered protein metabolism.

f. **Integumentary System**. Risk of skin breakdown, which leads to necrosis and ulceration of tissues, especially on bony areas.

g. **Urinary System**.

(1) Renal calculi (kidney stones) caused by stagnation of urine in the renal pelvis and the high levels of urinary calcium.

(2) Urinary tract infections caused by urinary stasis that favors the growth of bacteria.

(3) Decreased bladder muscle tone resulting in urinary retention.

h. **Metabolism**.

(1) Increased risk of electrolyte imbalance. An absence of weight on the skeleton and immobility causes protein to be broken down faster than it is made, resulting in a negative nitrogen balance.

(2) Decreased metabolic rate.

(3) Altered exchange of nutrients and gases.

i. **Psychosocial Functioning**.

(1) Decrease in self-concept and increase in sense of powerlessness due to inability to move purposefully and dependence on someone for assistance with simple self-care activities.

(2) Body image distortions (depends on diagnosis).

(3) Decrease in sensory stimulation due to lack of activity, and altered sleep-wake pattern.

(4) Increased risk of depression, which may cause the patient to become apathetic, possibly because of decreased sensory stimulation; or the patient may exhibit altered thought processes.

(5) Decreased social interaction.

## 5-3. THE PURPOSES OF EXERCISE FOR THE IMMOBILE PATIENT

a. To maintain joint mobility is done by putting each of the patient's joints through all possible movements to increase and/or maintain movement in each joint.

b. To prevent contracture, atony (insufficient muscular tone), and atrophy of muscles.

c. To stimulate circulation, preventing thrombus and embolus formation.

d. To improve coordination.

e. To increase tolerance for more activity.

f. To maintain and build muscle strength.

## 5-4. TYPES OF EXERCISES

a. **Passive.** These exercises are carried out by the nurse, without assistance from the patient. Passive exercises will not preserve muscle mass or bone mineralization because there is no voluntary contraction, lengthening of muscle, or tension on bones.

b. **Active Assistive**. These exercises are performed by the patient with assistance from the nurse. Active assistive exercises encourage normal muscle function while the nurse supports the distal joint.

c. **Active**. Active exercises are performed by the patient, without assistance, to increase muscle strength.

d. **Resistive**. These are active exercises performed by the patient by pulling or pushing against an opposing force.

e. **Isometric**. These exercises are performed by the patient by contracting and relaxing muscles while keeping the part in a fixed position. Isometric exercises are done to maintain muscle strength when a joint is immobilized. Full patient cooperation is required.

## 5-5. TYPES OF BODY MOVEMENT

**NOTE**: For types of body movement, see figure 5-1.

a. **Flexion**. The state of being bent. The cervical spine is flexed when the chin is moved toward the chest.

b. **Extension**. The state of being in a straight line. The cervical spine is extended when the head is held straight.

c. **Hyperextension**. The state of exaggerated extension. The cervical spine is hyperextended when the person looks overhead, toward the ceiling.

d. **Abduction**. Lateral movement of a body part away from the midline of the body. The arm is abducted when it is held away from the body.

e. **Adduction**. Lateral movement of a body part toward the midline of the body. The arm is adducted when it is moved from an outstretched position toward the body.

f. **Rotation**. Turning of a body part around an axis. The head is rotated when moved from side to side to indicate "no."

g. **Circumduction**. Rotating an extremity in a complete circle. Circumduction is a combination of abduction, adduction, extension, and flexion.

h. **Supination**. The palm or sole is rotated in an upward position

i. **Pronation**. The palm or sole is rotated in a downward position.

## 5-6. GUIDELINES FOR RANGE OF MOTION EXERCISES

a. Plan when range of motion exercises should be done (see figures 5-2 and 5-3). Plan whether exercises will be passive, active-assistive, or active. Involve the patient in planning the program of exercises and other activities because he/she will be more apt to do the exercises voluntarily.

b. Expect the patient's heart rate and respiratory rate to increase during exercise.

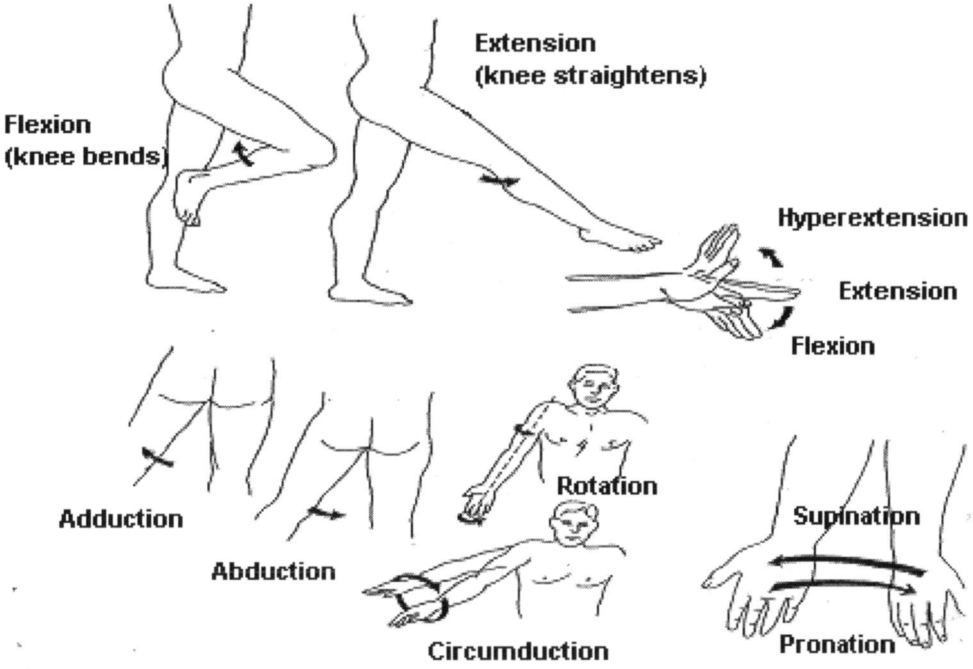


Figure 5-1. Types of body movement.

c. Range-of-motion exercises should be done at least twice a day. During the bath is one appropriate time. The warm bath water relaxes the muscles and decreases spasticity of the joints. Also, during the bath, areas are exposed so that the joints can be both moved and observed. Another appropriate time might be before bedtime. The joints of helpless or immobile patients should be exercised once every eight hours to prevent contracture from occurring.

d. Joints are exercised sequentially, starting with the neck and moving down. Put each joint needing exercise through the range of motion procedure a minimum of three times, and preferably five times. Avoid overexerting the patient; do not continue the exercises to the point that the patient develops fatigue. Some exercises may need to be delayed until the patient's condition improves.

ASSESSMENT/PLANNING RANGE OF MOTION EXERCISES

Patient ____________________ Page 1 of 2

Ward/Room/Bed/ ____________________

| ASSESSMENT | DATE | TIME | COMMENTS | INITIALS |
|---|---|---|---|---|
| 1. Assess joint mobility and activity status. | | | | |
| 2. Assess general health status. | | | | |
| 3. Assess patient's ability to participate. | | | | |
| **PLANNING** | | | | |
| 4. Plan time for exercises. | | | | |
| 5. Plan type of exercises. | | | | |

Figure 5-2. Example of Assessment/Planning Form.

e. Start gradually and move slowly using smooth and rhythmic movements appropriate for the patient's condition.

f. Support the extremity when giving passive exercise to the joints of the arm or leg.

g. Stretch the muscles and keep the joint flexible.

h. Move each joint until there is resistance, but never force a joint to the point of pain.

i. Keep friction at a minimum to avoid injuring the skin.

j. Return the joint to its neutral position.

k. Use passive exercises as required, however, encourage active exercises when the patient is able to do so.

FLOW SHEET - RANGE OF MOTION EXERCISES

Patient ______________________ Page 2 of 2

Ward/Room/Bed/ ____________________ Date ______________

| MOVEMENT | TIME | | | COMMENTS |
|---|---|---|---|---|
| | 0900 | 1700 | | |
| *R Upper Extremity* | | | | |
| *Shoulder flexion* | ✓ | | | |
| *Shoulder external rotation* | ✓ | | | |
| *Elbow extension* | ✓ | | | *limited to 120°* |
| *Wrist extension* | ✓ | | | |
| *Finger extension* | ✓ | | | |
| *R Lower Extremity* | | | | |
| *Hip abduction* | ✓ | | | |
| *Hip extension* | ✓ | | | |
| *Knee extension* | ✓ | | | |
| *Ankle dorsiflexion* | ✓ | | | |
| NURSE'S INITIALS | *JHS* | | | |

Figure 5-3. Range of Motion Flow Sheet

## 5-7. DOCUMENTATION

a. **Evaluation.** Evaluate the patient in terms of fatigue, joint discomfort, and joint mobility.

b. **Record Keeping**. Range of motion is often placed on a flow sheet (see figure 5-3). If a flow sheet is not used, an entry should be made in the Nursing Progress Notes using a narrative format. If there is any adverse response to the exercises, a narrative note must be made. Nursing notes should address the extent to which joints can be moved in degrees (see figure 5-4).

| Date/Time | Nursing Progress Notes |
|---|---|
| *9 Oct 92* | *Passive ROM performed after bedbath. Extension of arm at elbow* |
| *0900* | *limited to approximately 120˚. J. Sanders, LVN* |
| | |
| | |
| | |

Figure 5-4. Example of Narrative Note.

## 5-8. CONTRAINDICATIONS TO RANGE OF MOTION EXERCISES

a. **Heart and Respiratory Diseases**. Range of motion exercises require energy and tend to increase circulation. Increasing the level of energy expended or increasing the demand for circulation is potentially hazardous to patients with heart and respiratory diseases.

b. **Connective Tissue Disorders**. Range of motion exercises put stress on the soft tissues of the joint and on the bony structures. These exercises should not be performed if the joints are swollen or inflamed or if there has been injury to the musculoskeletal system in the vicinity of the joint.

## 5-9. CLOSING

Encourage the immobile patient to participate as fully as possible so that he feels involved in the process. Always explain to the patient what you are about to do and enlist his cooperation. To avoid strain, remember to maintain your own proper body mechanics as you carry out the exercises for the patient. The overall nursing goal is to promote the maximum degree of mobility for the patient who cannot engage in the normal activities of daily living and prevent or reduce the effects of immobility. Performing range of motion exercises can often save the patient a lengthy rehabilitation.

***Continue with Exercises***

## EXERCISES, LESSON 5

**INSTRUCTIONS**. The following exercises are to be answered by completing the incomplete statement or by writing the answer in the space provided at the end of the question.

After you have completed all the exercises, turn to "Solutions to Exercises" at the end of the lesson and check your answers.

1. Regular exercise contributes to a healthy body. Immobility has a __________ effect.

2. When a joint cannot be moved and exercised through normal activities of daily living, the patient or nurse must move it at regular intervals to maintain ______________ and ______________________.

3. Range of motion exercises are ones in which a nurse or patient moves each joint. ______________________________________________.

4. The effects of immobility on the cardiac system include:

   a. ______________________________.

   b. ______________________________.

   c. ______________________________.

   d. ______________________________.

5. The effects of immobility on the respiratory system include:

   a. ______________________________.

   b. ______________________________.

   c. ______________________________.

6. The effects of immobility on the musculoskeletal system include:

   a. ______________________________.

   b. ______________________________.

   c. ______________________________.

   d. ______________________________.

7. The effects of immobility on the nervous system include:

   a. ______________________________.

   b. ______________________________.

8. The effects of immobility on the gastrointestinal system include:

   a. ______________________________.

   b. ______________________________.

9. One effect of immobility on the integumentary system is ______________________________.

10. An absence of weight bearing on the skeleton and immobility causes protein to be broken down faster than it is made, resulting in a ____________________.

11. The inability to move purposefully and dependence on someone for assistance with simple self-care activities results in a decrease in and an increase in a ________________________________________.

12. Four purposes of exercise for the immobile patient are:

a. ______________________________.

b. ______________________________.

c. ______________________________.

d. ______________________________.

13. The five types of exercises are:

a. ______________________________.

b. ______________________________.

c. ______________________________.

d. ______________________________.

e. ______________________________.

14. The nine types of body movement are:

a. ______________________________.

b. ______________________________.

c. ______________________________.

d. ______________________________.

f. ______________________________.

g. ______________________________.

h. ______________________________.

i. ______________________________.

15. Range of motion exercises should be done at least ____________________. The joints of helpless or immobile patients should be exercised once every ____________________ to prevent contracture.

16. Joints should be exercised sequentially, starting with the____________ and moving ___________.

17. Each joint needing exercise should be put through the range of motion procedure a minimum of _________________________.

18. One guideline for range of motion exercises is to move each joint until there is _________________ but never force a joint to the point of ______________.

19. When documenting that range of motion exercises have been done, the nurse should evaluate the patient in terms of:

a. _____________________________.

b. _____________________________.

c. _____________________________.

20. If there is any adverse response to the exercises, a____________________ must be made.

21. Two contraindications to range of motion exercises are:

a. ___________________________.

b. ___________________________.

***Check Your Answers on Next Page***

**SOLUTIONS TO EXERCISES, LESSON 5**

1. Negative. (para 5-1)

2. Muscles tone, joint mobility. (para 5-1)

3. Through as full a range as possible without causing pain. (para 5-1)

4. Venous stasis.
Increased cardiac workload.
Thrombus and embolus formation.
Orthostatic hypotension. (paras 5-2a(1)--(4))

5. Hypostatic pneumonia.
Atelectasis.
Impaired coughing mechanism. (paras 5-2b(1)--(3))

6. Muscle atrophy.
Contracture.
Ankylosis.
Osteoporosis. (paras 5-2c(1)--(4))

7. Altered sensation.
Peripheral nerve palsy. (paras 5-2d(1), (2))

8. Disturbance in appetite.
Altered digestion and utilization of nutrients.
Altered protein metabolism. (paras 5-2e(1)--(3))

9. Risk of skin breakdown. (para 5-2f)

10. Negative nitrogen balance. (para 5-2h(1))

11. Self concept, sense of powerlessness. (para 5-2i(1))

12. (Any four of the following):

To maintain joint mobility.
To prevent contracture, atony, and atrophy of muscles.
To prevent thrombus and embolus formation.
To improve coordination.
To increase tolerance for more activity.
To maintain and build muscle strength. (para 5-3--f)

13. Passive.
    Active assistive.
    Active.
    Resistive.
    Isometric. (paras 5-4a--e)

14. Flexion.
    Extension.
    Hyperextension.
    Abduction.
    Adduction.
    Rotation.
    Circumduction.
    Supination.
    Pronation. (paras 5-5a--i)

15. Twice a day, eight hours. (para 5-6c)

16. Neck, down. (5-6d)

17. Three times. (Para 5-6d)

18. Resistance, pain. (para 5-6h)

19. Fatigue.
    Joint discomfort.
    Joint mobility. (para 5-7a)

20. Narrative note. (para 5-7b, figure 5-4)

21. Heart and respiratory diseases.
    Connective tissue disorders. (paras 5-8a, b)

END OF LESSON 3

## LESSON ASSIGNMENT

| | |
|---|---|
| **LESSON 6** | Environmental Health and the Practical Nurse. |
| **LESSON ASSIGNMENT** | Paragraphs 6-1 through 6-5. |
| **LESSON OBJECTIVES** | After completing this lesson, you should be able to: |
| | 6-1. Select the hospital electrical safety measures when given a list of safety measures. |
| | 6-2. Select the hospital fire safety measures when given a list of safety measures. |
| | 6-3. Select the safety measures which pertain to the patient care environment. |
| **SUGGESTION**: | After studying the assignment, complete the exercises at the end of this lesson. These exercises will help you to achieve the lesson objectives. |

# LESSON 6

# ENVIRONMENTAL HEALTH AND THE PRACTICAL NURSE

## 6-1. INTRODUCTION

One of the most important aspects of patient care is to ensure safety for each patient throughout the day. It is impossible to prevent accidents completely. However, there are ways to limit the potential for accidents that may cause injury to the patient or health care personnel and the unnecessary loss of equipment.

## 6-2. HOSPITAL ELECTRICAL SAFETY MEASURES

a. Use electrical equipment for the intended purpose only.

b. Keep television sets, telephones, radios, hair dryers, electric shavers, and all other electrical equipment and appliances away from bathtubs and washbasins.

c. Test all small appliances before use to see that they are in good working order. Ensure periodic service checks of all electrical equipment.

d. Remove a plug from a wall socket by grasping the plug, not the cord.

e. Use plugs and outlets with a ground when possible. Do not overload an electrical outlet.

f. Do not kink electric cords; this may cause the fine wires inside the cord to break.

g. Never use faulty equipment. If an appliance overheats, produces a shock or gives off an odor while being used, remove the appliance from the area. Follow procedures to have the appliance evaluated by medical maintenance.

**NOTE:** An electric spark near a high concentration of oxygen or certain anesthetic gases may cause an instant and serious fire.

## 6-3. HOSPITAL FIRE SAFETY MEASURES

a. Despite the use of fire retardant material, and compliance with fire regulations, fires still occur. Health care facilities should have regular fire drills so that all personnel know exactly what to do. Health care personnel should be trained and drilled in:

(1) Fire prevention.

(2) Location and use of fire alarms.

(3) Location and use of fire extinguishers.

(4) Location of emergency exits.

(5) Evacuation procedures.

b. Oxygen supports combustion. Post signs to show that oxygen is in use where applicable. If a patient is receiving oxygen as part of his treatment, be sure that the patient, his roommates, and visitors know that smoking is prohibited.

**NOTE**: Smoking is prohibited in treatment areas of most health care facilities.

c. If a fire occurs, follow these steps:

(1) Activate the fire alarm procedures.

(2) Turn off oxygen, lights, and any electrical equipment in the vicinity of the fire.

(3) Remove the patients who are in immediate danger.

(4) Notify the hospital "switchboard" of the location of the fire.

(6) Close windows and doors to reduce ventilation.

(5) Using the fire extinguisher, attempt to extinguish the fire.

(7) Return patients who are not endangered to their rooms.

(8) Post a guard to direct the fire department.

## 6-4. PATIENT CARE ENVIRONMENT SAFETY MEASURES

a. Identify patients at risk for injury. Those at special risk include:

(1) Elderly or confused patients.

(2) Patients with impaired vision or hearing.

(3) Patients with impaired mobility (wheelchairs, walkers, and partial paralysis).

(4) Patients with a history of falls.

(5) Patients with a history of substance abuse.

(6) Patients receiving medication that interferes with reasoning or motor functions.

b. Protect the patients at risk for injury.

c. To prevent falls:

(1) Place the bed in the low position.

(2) Keep the side rails up when the patient is not receiving bedside care.

(3) Advise the patient to wear low-heeled shoes that fit well when walking.

(4) Ensure that nonskid strips or mats are affixed to the bottom of bathtubs and shower floors.

(5) Ensure that bathtubs have sturdy handrails and shower stools are in place when needed.

(6) Warn patients and visitors when floors are wet and slippery. Also see that signs are posted.

d. Protective restraints (see figures 6-1 through 6-3).

(1) Use restraints when careful assessment indicates that these are needed. (Some facilities require a doctor's order for restraints).

(2) Movement is essential to the patient's well being. Use the least restrictive type of restraint, which will protect the patient.

(3) Apply the restraint for the shortest amount of time necessary. The vest restraint (figure 6-2) may only be necessary while a patient is sitting in a wheelchair.

(4) Provide for as much movement as possible. The waist restraint (figure 6-3) protects the patient from falling out of bed but still allows the patient to change position independently.

(5) Restrain the fewest limbs or body parts possible. However, if leg restraints are necessary, use wrist restraints also. If this is not done, the patient may remove the leg restraints or he may accidentally hang by his heels in the restraints.

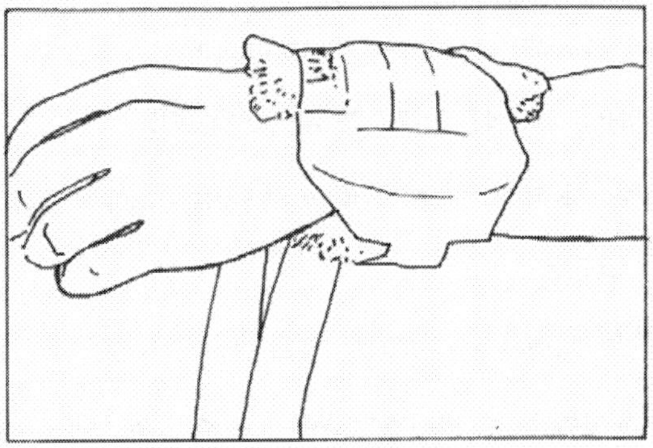

Figure 6-1. Wrist of ankle restraint.

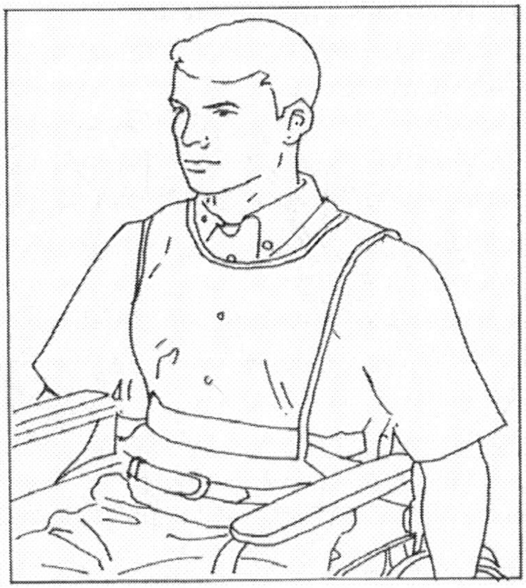

Figure 6-2. Vest restraint.

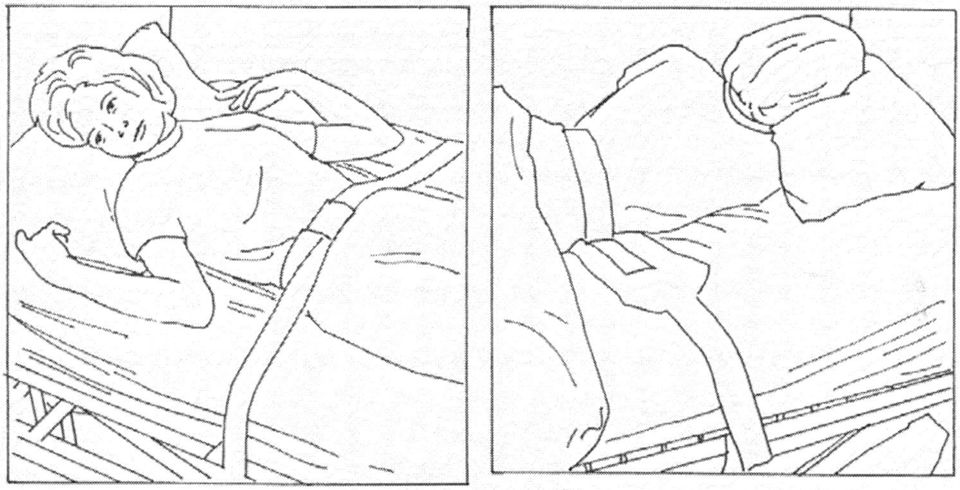

Figure 6-3. Waist restraint.

(6) Tie the restraint with a knot that is not likely to come loose, yet can be released easily by the nurse in an emergency. A half-bow knot (figure 6-4) meets these criteria.

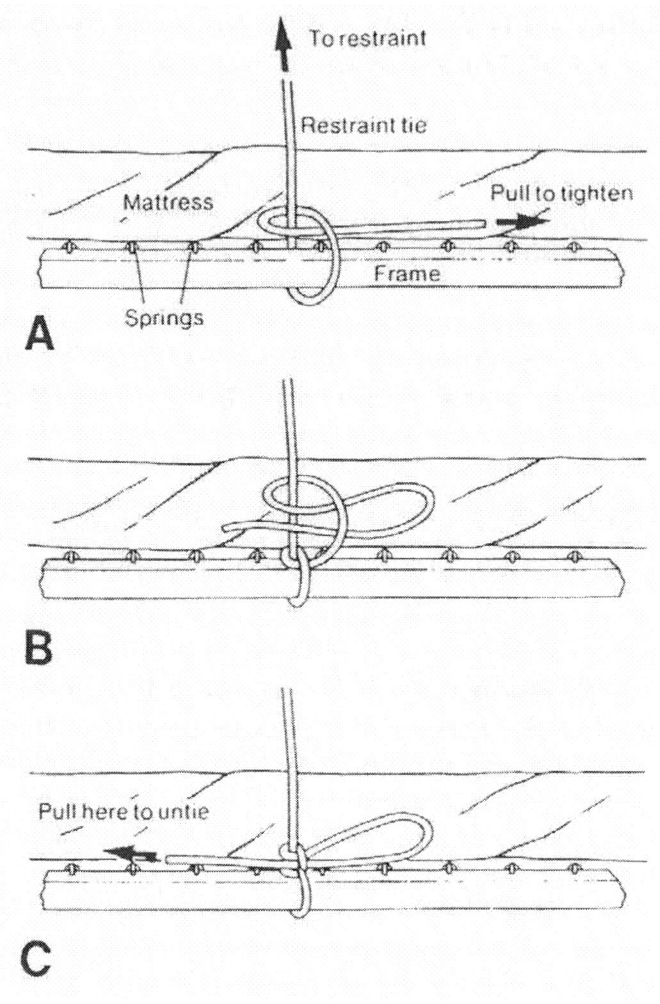


Figure 6-4. Half-bow knot.

(7) Explain to the patient the reason for the restraint. Position him comfortably and change his position every 2 hours. Feed the patient who must remain restrained during meals. Help him use the toilet, bedpan, or urinal at regular intervals.

e. Prevent scalds and burns.

(1) Place coffee, tea, and other hot liquids where the patient can reach them easily and safely.

(2) Assist the patient if there is any doubt about whether he can safely regulate the temperature of water in tubs or showers.

(3) Carefully follow policy when using hot-water bags or heating pads. Because of the danger of burning patients, many health care facilities do not allow their use.

f. Prevent the spread of infection. A health care facility may adopt its own infection control policies and practices. However, the procedures generally follow the recommendations from the Centers for Disease Control (CDC). This is a federal agency that studies pathogens, outbreaks of contagious diseases, and methods used to control these outbreaks.

(1) Preventing disease, including infections, is a high priority in health care. Nurses should use techniques that prevent microorganisms from living, growing, and spreading.

(2) Two methods are used to reduce or eliminate the presence of microorganisms and thus prevent infections. These two methods are called surgical asepsis and medical asepsis.

(a) Surgical asepsis refers to the practice that eliminates the presence of all microorganisms (bacteria, viruses, fungi, yeasts, molds, rickettsia, and protozoa). This practice is sterilization.

(b) Medical asepsis refers to practices that help reduce the number and inhibit the growth of microorganisms, especially pathogens (those that cause infections or contagious diseases). Medical asepsis, also called clean technique includes use of antimicrobial agents, hand washing, cleaning supplies and equipment, and disinfection.

(3) Infections and infectious diseases begin in a reservoir and move full circle to a susceptible host (see figure 6-5).

(a) Reservoir. This is the place on which or in which organisms grow and reproduce. Examples include man and animals.

(b) Exit from reservoir. Escape routes for organisms include the nose, throat, mouth, ear, eye, intestinal tract, urinary tract, and wounds.

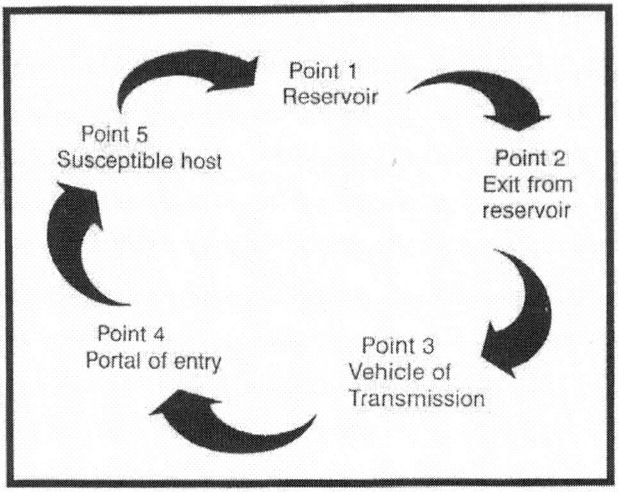


Figure 6-5. The infectious process cycle.

(c) Vehicle of transmission. The means by which organisms are carried about include hands, equipment, instruments, china and silverware, linens, and droplets.

(d) Portal of entry. The part of the body where organisms enter include any break in skin or mucous membrane, the mouth, nose, and genitourinary tract.

(e) Susceptible host. A person who cannot fight off the organism once it enters his body and therefore, he becomes ill.

(4) It is important that the nurse teach patients facts and practices about surgical and medical asepsis. When teaching a patient you should:

(a) Observe the patient to identify areas where instruction would be helpful in controlling the spread of infection.

(b) Act as a model by using sound practices of asepsis when giving care.

(c) Provide guidance to the patient who must give himself care at home in the proper way to handle sterile equipment and supplies and in how to sterilize reusable items.

g. Report infections. Health care workers must report any infection that occurs. The Infection Control Committee will investigate any case of infection to determine the cause. If a break in nursing technique is identified, the committee will propose different procedures to eliminate the problem.

## 6-5. CLOSING

Maslow states that our safety and security needs are second only to the need for food, air, and water. The daily responsibility for protecting the patient from additional injury or illness rests with the nursing team. The skillful and knowledgeable nurse can be just as dangerous as the incompetent one if safety measures are not applied in the health care environment.

***Continue with Exercises***

## EXERCISES, LESSON 6

**INSTRUCTION**: Answer the following exercises by marking the lettered response that best answers the exercise, by completing the statement, or by writing the answer in the space provided at the end of the exercise.

After you have completed all of these exercises, turn to "Solutions to Exercises" at the end of the lesson and check your answers. For each exercise answered incorrectly, reread the material referenced with the solution.

1. One of the most important aspects of patient care is ____________________

   ________________________________________.

2. Electrical appliances should be used for ________________________________ only.

3. Before use __________ all small appliances to see that they are in good working order.

4. When removing an electrical plug from a wall socket, grasp _________________

5. Kinking an electric cord may cause ____________________________________.

6. If an appliance overheats, produces a shock, or gives off an odor while being used, ______________________________________________________________.

7. Health care personnel should be trained and drilled in:

   a. ___________________________________.

   b. ___________________________________.

   c. ___________________________________.

   d. ___________________________________.

   e. ___________________________________.

8. If a patient is receiving oxygen as part of his treatment, be sure that he, his roommates, and visitors know that _______________is prohibited.

9. If a fire occurs, hospital personnel should turn off __________, ___________, and _______________________________ in the vicinity of the fire.

10. If a fire occurs, you should notify the ___________________ of the location of the fire and______________________ to direct the fire department.

11. Safety measures which pertain to the patient care environment include identifying ___________________________________________________________.

12. Patients at special risk for injury include:

    a. _________________________________.

    b. _________________________________.

    c. _________________________________.

    d. _________________________________.

    e. _________________________________.

    f. _________________________________.

13. To prevent falls, you should place the bed in the ________, position and keep the ___________ up.

14. To prevent falls, you should ensure that ___________________or _________ are affixed to the bottom of bathtubs and shower floors.

15. Some health care facilities require a _______________________ for use of protective restraints.

16. Because movement is essential to the patient's well being, you should use the ________________________ type of restraint, which will protect the patient.

17. You should apply a protective restraint for the ________________ amount of time necessary.

18. When using protective restraints, provide as much movement as possible. The _______________________ protects the patient from falling out of bed but still allows the patient to change positions.

19. If leg restraints are necessary to protect the patient, you should use __________ _______________ also.

20. Two methods are used to reduce or eliminate the presence of microorganisms and thus prevent infections. These two methods are:

    a. ________________________.

    b. ________________________.

21. _______________________ refers to the practice that eliminates the presence of all microorganisms.

22. _______________________ refers to the practices that help reduce the number and inhibit the growth of microorganisms.

23. Infections and infectious diseases begin in a __________________and moves full circle to a _________________________

24. Portals of entry for microorganisms that cause infections and infectious diseases include:

    a. _______________________________.

    b. _______________________________.

    c. _______________________________.

    d. _______________________________.

    e. _______________________________.

25. It is important that the nurse teach patients about surgical and medical asepsis. When doing so, you should:

a.______________________________________________.

b.______________________________________________.

c.______________________________________________.

***Check Your Answers on Next Page***

**SOLUTIONS TO EXERCISES, LESSON 6**

1. To ensure safety for each patient. (para 6-1)

2. The intended purpose. (para 6-2a)

3. Test. (para 6-2c)

4. The plug. (para 6-2d)

5. The fine wires inside the cord to break. (para 6-2f)

6. Remove the appliance from the area. (para 6-2g)

7. Fire prevention.
   Location and use of fire alarms.
   Location and use of fire extinguishers.
   Location of emergency exits.
   Evacuation procedures. (paras 6-3a(1)--(5))

8. Smoking. (para 6-3b)

9. Oxygen, lights, any electrical equipment. (para 6-3c(2))

10. Switchboard, post a guard. (paras 6-3c(4), (8))

11. Patients at risk for injury. (para 6-4a)

12. Elderly or confused patients.
    Patients with impaired vision or hearing.
    Patients with impaired mobility.
    Patients with a history of falls.
    Patients with a history of substance abuse.
    Patients receiving medications that interfere with reasoning or motor functions.
    (paras 6-4a(1)--(6))

13. Low, side rails. (paras 6-4c(1), (2))

14. Nonskid strips, mats. (para 6-4c(4))

15. A doctor's order. (para 6-4d(1))

16. Least restrictive. (para 6-4d(2))

17. Shortest. (para 6-4d(3))

18. Waist restraint. (para 6-4d(4))

19. Arm restraints. (para 6-4d(5))

20. Surgical asepsis.
    Medical asepsis. (paras 6-4f(1). (2))

21. Surgical asepsis. (para 6-4f(2)(a))

22. Medical asepsis. (para 6-4f(2)(b))

23. Reservoir, susceptible host. (para 6-4f(3))

24. Break in skin.
    Mucous membranes.
    The mouth.
    The nose.
    The genitourinary tract. (para 6-4f(3)(d))

25. Observe the patient to identify areas where instruction would be helpful in controlling the spread of infection.

    Act as a model by using sound practices of asepsis when giving care.

    Provide guidance in practices of asepsis to the patient who must give himself care at home. (paras 6-4f(4)(a)--(c))

***END OF LESSON 6***

# COMMENT SHEET

## SUBCOURSE MD0905, Nursing Fundamentals I — EDITION 100

Your comments about this subcourse are valuable and aid the writers in refining the subcourse and making it more usable. Please enter your comments in the space provided. ENCLOSE THIS FORM (OR A COPY) WITH YOUR ANSWER SHEET **ONLY** IF YOU HAVE COMMENTS ABOUT THIS SUBCOURSE..

**FOR A WRITTEN REPLY, WRITE A SEPARATE LETTER AND INCLUDE SOCIAL SECURITY NUMBER, RETURN ADDRESS (and e-mail address, if possible), SUBCOURSE NUMBER AND EDITION, AND PARAGRAPH/EXERCISE/EXAMINATION ITEM NUMBER.**

## PLEASE COMPLETE THE FOLLOWING ITEMS:

(Use the reverse side of this sheet, if necessary.)

1. List any terms that were not defined properly.

2. List any errors.

   paragraph    error    correction

3. List any suggestions you have to improve this subcourse.

4. Student Information (optional)

Name/Rank ____________
SSN ____________
Address ____________
E mail Address ____________
Telephone number (DSN) ____________
MOS/AOC ____________

**PRIVACY ACT STATEMENT (AUTHORITY: 10USC3012(B) AND (G))**

**PURPOSE:** To provide Army Correspondence Course Program students a means to submit inquiries and comments.

**USES:** To locate and make necessary change to student records.

**DISCLOSURE:** **VOLUNTARY.** Failure to submit SSN will prevent subcourse authors at service school from accessing student records and responding to inquiries requiring such follow-ups.

U.S. ARMY MEDICAL DEPARTMENT CENTER AND SCHOOL    Fort Sam Houston, Texas 78234 6130

# Nursing Fundamentals II

# Subcourse MD0906

This page intentionally left blank.

U.S. ARMY MEDICAL DEPARTMENT CENTER AND SCHOOL
FORT SAM HOUSTON, TEXAS 78234-6100

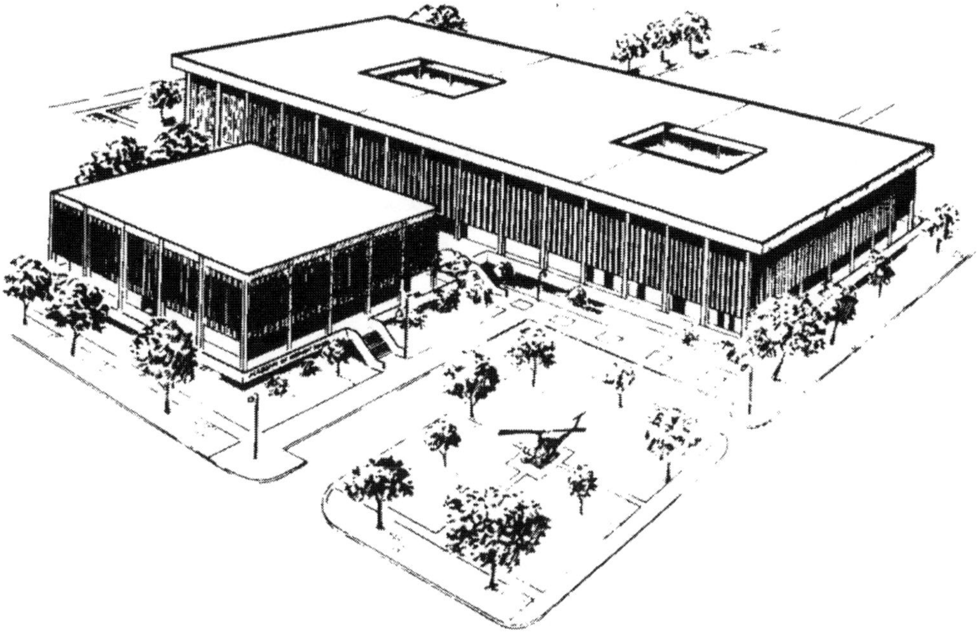

# NURSING FUNDAMENTALS II

## SUBCOURSE MD0906 EDITION 100

## DEVELOPMENT

This subcourse is approved for resident and correspondence course instruction. It reflects the current thought of the Academy of Health Sciences and conforms to printed Department of the Army doctrine as closely as currently possible. Development and progress render such doctrine continuously subject to change.

## ADMINISTRATION

For comments or questions regarding enrollment, student records, or shipments, contact the Nonresident Instruction Section at DSN 471-5877, commercial (210) 221-5877, toll-free 1-800-344-2380; fax: 210-221-4012 or DSN 471-4012, e-mail accp@amedd.army.mil, or write to:

COMMANDER
AMEDDC&S
ATTN MCCS HSN
2105 11TH STREET SUITE 4192
FORT SAM HOUSTON TX 78234-5064

Approved students whose enrollments remain in good standing may apply to the Nonresident Instruction Section for subsequent courses by telephone, letter, or e-mail.

Be sure your social security number is on all correspondence sent to the Academy of Health Sciences.

## CLARIFICATION OF TRAINING LITERATURE TERMINOLOGY

When used in this publication, words such as "he," "him," "his," and "men" are intended to include both the masculine and feminine genders, unless specifically stated otherwise or when obvious in context.

**TABLE OF CONTENTS**

**CORRESPONDENCE COURSE OF THE**
**U.S. ARMY MEDICAL DEPARTMENT CENTER AND SCHOOL**

## SUBCOURSE MD0906

## NURSING FUNDAMENTALS II

## INTRODUCTION

As a member of the health-care team, the practical nurse participates in assessing the patient's physical status, in meeting the patient's nutritional needs, in preparing the patient for diagnostic and surgical procedures, and in teaching the patient self-care.

This subcourse will present theory and concepts that the practical nurse should know in order to assist in patient evaluation and function as a team leader in the health-care environment.

Subcourse Components:

This subcourse consists of 8 lessons. The lessons are:

Lesson 1. Assisting with the Physical Examination.

Lesson 2. Specimen Collection.

Lesson 3. Catheterization of the Male and Female Patient.

Lesson 4. Vital Signs.

Lesson 5. Diet Therapy.

Lesson 6. Introduction to Physical Assessment.

Lesson 7. The Role of the Practical Nurse.

Lesson 8. Perioperative Patient Care.

Study Suggestions:

Here are some suggestions that may be helpful to you in completing this subcourse:

--Read and study each lesson carefully.

--Complete the subcourse lesson by lesson. After completing each lesson, work the exercises at the end of the lesson, marking your answers in this booklet.

--After completing each set of lesson exercises, compare your answers with those on the solution sheet that follows the exercises. If you have answered an exercise incorrectly, check the reference cited after the answer on the solution sheet to determine why your response was not the correct one.

Credit Awarded:

To receive credit hours, you must be officially enrolled and complete an examination furnished by the Nonresident Instruction Section at Fort Sam Houston, Texas. Upon successful completion of the examination for this subcourse, you will be awarded 12 credit hours.

You can enroll by going to the web site http://atrrs.army.mil and enrolling under "Self Development" (School Code 555).

A listing of correspondence courses and subcourses available through the Nonresident Instruction Section is found in Chapter 4 of DA Pamphlet 350-59, Army Correspondence Course Program Catalog. The DA PAM is available at the following website: http://www.usapa.army.mil/pdffiles/p350-59.pdf.

# STANDARD PRECAUTIONS

## Prevention of Transmission of Human Immunodeficiency Virus and Other Blood-Borne Pathogens in Health Care Settings

Only blood, semen, vaginal secretions, and possibly breast milk have been implicated in transmission of human immunodeficiency virus (HIV), hepatitis B virus (HBV), and other blood-borne pathogens.

Blood is the single most important source of transmission of blood-borne pathogens in health care settings. Infection control efforts must focus on preventing exposures to blood.

Although the risk is unknown, standard precautions also apply to tissues and to cerebrospinal fluid, synovial fluid, pleural fluid, peritoneal fluid, and amniotic fluid. Sta precautions do not apply to feces, nasal secretions, sputum, sweat, tears, urine, and vomitus unless they contain visible blood. Although standard precautions do not apply to these body substances, the wise nurse wears gloves for protection from other infections.

Precautions are used for *all* patients. (*Reason:* It is impossible to know which patients are infected with such conditions as HIV, HBV, or other infectious agents.)

Gloves are worn *whenever* the health care worker may come in contact with blood, body fluids containing blood, and other body fluids to which standard precautions apply. (*Reason:* Diseases can be carried in the body substances.)

Wear gloves *at all times* if you have any break in the skin of your hands. If you have an exudative condition, such as weeping dermatitis, you must be evaluated before working with patients and patient care equipment. (*Reason:* You may be at great risk of contracting a disease; you might also spread disease.)

Change gloves after each contact with a client. (*Reason:* The gloves may be contaminated.)

Wash your hands and skin surfaces immediately and thoroughly if they are contaminated with blood or body fluids. (*Reason:* Proper washing will help to stop the spread of infection.)

Wear a gown or apron when clothing could become soiled. (*Reason:* To prevent spread of infection to yourself or others.)

Wear a mask and eye protection if splashing is possible. Hospital protocol will determine what type of eye protection is required for each specific case. (*Reason:* Infection could enter your body through the mucous membranes of your mouth or nose or through your eyes.)

Dispose of sharp objects carefully. Do not recap or break needles. Needles and sharp objects are placed in a special container after use. (*Reason:* There is a possibility of accidental finger stick. It is important to protect yourself and housekeeping personnel.)

If you have an on-the-job accident that causes a break in the skin, notify your nursing supervisor *immediately*. (*Reason:* Immediate precautions must be taken to protect you.)

Special care is taken of a deceased patient's body. (*Reason:* To prevent leakage of body substances. It is safer to assume that all patients are infectious.)

All health care workers who perform or assist in vaginal or cesarean delivery should wear gloves and gowns when handling the placenta or the infant until blood and amniotic fluid have been removed from the infant's skin. Gloves should be worn until after postdelivery care of the umbilical cord.

Pregnant health care workers are not known to be at greater risk of contracting HIV infection than health care workers who are not pregnant; however, if a health care worker develops HIV infection during pregnancy, the infant is at risk. Because of this risk, pregnant health care workers should be especially familiar with and strictly adhere to precautions to minimize the risk of HIV transmission.

*(Adapted from Centers for Disease Control: Recommendations for prevention of HIV transmission in health care settings. MMWR 36: Suppl. 25: 1987. Centers for Disease Control: Update: Standard precautions for prevention or transmission of human immunodeficiency virus, hepatitis B virus, and other blood-borne pathogens in health-care settings. MMWR 37: 24, 1988)*

***End of Standard Precautions***

## LESSON ASSIGNMENT

**LESSON 1** Assisting With The Physical Examination

**TEXT ASSIGNMENT** Paragraphs 1-1 through 1-10

**LESSON OBJECTIVES** After completing this lesson, you should be able to:
Select the purposes for performing a physical examination.

1-2. Select the functions of the practical nurse during the physical examination.

1-3. Identify the health care providers who could perform the physical examination.

1-4. Identify the body systems that the health care provider would usually examine during a physical examination.

1-5. Select the physiological measurements/ values which are routinely made during a complete physical examination.

1-6. Identify the supplies and equipment that should be available in the examination room.

1-7. Select the nursing implications, which apply during the physical examination of a patient.

1-8. Match the correct body position with the description or an illustration of the body position.

1-9. Select the purposes for draping a patient during the physical examination.

1-10. Select the nursing implications, which relate to evaluation of the patient's condition in terms of the need for assistance during a physical examination.

**SUGGESTION** After studying the assignment, complete the exercises at the end of this lesson. These exercises will help you to achieve the lesson objectives.

# LESSON 1

# ASSISTING WITH THE PHYSICAL EXAMINATION

## 1-1. INTRODUCTION

The history and the physical exam provide much of the information known about the patient's health status. As a practical nurse, you may be called upon to assist the physician or other health care providers during a physical examination. You should know the basics of the examination in order to have the appropriate equipment and supplies on hand, and so that you may place the patient in the proper position and drape him correctly.

## 1-2. PURPOSES FOR PERFORMING A PHYSICAL EXAMINATION

The physical examination can be performed by the following health care providers: a physician, nurse practitioner, or physician assistant. The health care provider makes specific and general observations as he examines the patient from head to toe. The exam should include the eyes, ears, nose, mouth, throat, neck, chest, breasts, abdomen, and extremities. A vaginal or rectal examination is performed if indicated. The purposes for performing a physical examination are:

a. To determine the patient's level of health or physiological function.

b. To arrive at a tentative diagnosis when there is a health problem or disease.

c. To confirm a diagnosis of disease or dysfunction.

d. To evaluate the effectiveness of prescribed medical treatment and therapy.

## 1-3. FUNCTIONS OF THE PRACTICAL NURSE DURING THE EXAMINATION PROCEDURE

a. Ensure that the patient feels comfortable and is not embarrassed. Prior to the examination, tell the patient what will take place and explain the reason for the procedure. The patient who knows what to expect will be more relaxed and cooperative.

b. Ask the patient to void into a urine specimen cup in order to empty the bladder and save the urine specimen for urinalysis. Have the patient put on a hospital gown so that his body is more accessible for examination.

c. Arrange equipment and supplies. Be sure that you have <u>everything</u> needed (see Table 1-1). Test all equipment to make certain that it works correctly.

| Supplies and Equipment |
| --- |
| Hospital gown<br>Sheet or disposable paper drapes<br>Bath blanket (to prevent chill)<br>Tray with flashlight, gloves, lubricant normal saline, cotton-tipped applicators, and tissues<br>Basin for soiled instruments<br>Waste container for paper goods<br>Scale with height measuring rod<br>Gooseneck lamp or hospital light<br>Gloves<br>Thermometer (oral or rectal)<br>Tape measure<br>Tongue depressors<br>Ophthalmoscope (for examining eyes)<br>Otoscope (for examining ears)<br>Tuning fork<br>Blood pressure apparatus and stethoscope<br>Percussion hammer (to check reflexes)<br>Red and blue pencils (to mark skin)<br>Small speculum (for nose examination)<br>Head mirror (to reflect light into body orifice, such as the throat<br><br>You may also need slides, blood tubes, a vaginal speculum, or other equipment; medications; and a surgical permit if a biopsy or other tests are to be done. |

Table 1-1. Supplies and equipment.

d. Accompany the patient to the examination room and assist him onto the table. Your presence lends support and reassurance to the patient. If a male is examining a female patient, or vice versa, stay in the room to protect the patient, the health care provider, and the hospital or clinic.

e. Wash your hands and measure the patient's vital signs (temperature, pulse, respiration, blood pressure), height, and weight. Wear gloves if the patient has a draining wound, is bleeding, is vomiting, or has an infection. (See Standard Precautions in this subcourse).

f. Have the patient's chart available. The physician needs to know the information that has already been obtained via the nursing observations and lab reports. Call the physician's attention to any abnormal lab values. Do this away from the patient.

g. Have all lab slips and x-ray slips ready with the patient's name, rank, social security number, date, and other required information.

h. Assist the patient to assume the proper position for each part of the examination (see figures 1-1 to 1-7). To provide continuing privacy, be sure to adjust the drapes each time the patient assumes a different position. If the patient is asked to stand erect, place paper towels on the floor or have the patient put on slippers.

i. Hand instruments and supplies to the physician. Properly label and care for all specimens collected.

j. See that the patient is returned safely to his room and is comfortable.

k. Place all instruments in the proper area for disinfection or sterilization and dispose of all wastes. Wash your hands again. See that the examination room is cleaned. Decontaminate the room if necessary. Change the cover on the tables. Replace all equipment.

## 1-4. POSITIONING A PATIENT FOR EXAMINATION OR TREATMENT

Patients are put in special positions for examination, for treatment or test, and to obtain specimens. You should know the positions used, how to assist the patient, and how to adjust the drapes.

a. **Horizontal Recumbent Position**. Used for most physical examinations. Patient is on his back with legs extended. Arms may be above the head, alongside the body or folded on the chest.

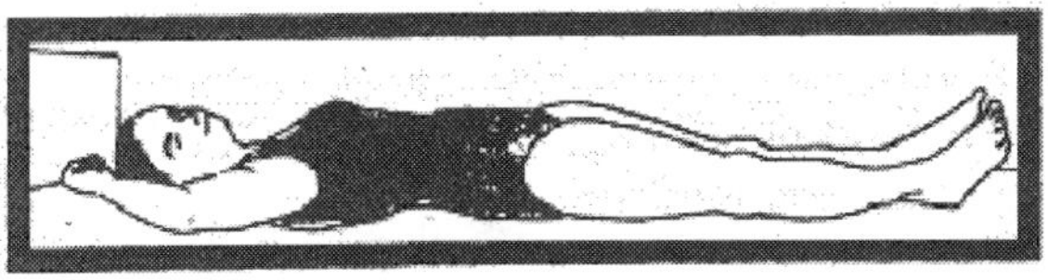

Figure 1-1. Horizontal recumbent position.

b. **Dorsal Recumbent Position**. Patient is on his back with knees flexed and soles of feet flat on the bed. Fold sheet once across the chest. Fold a second sheet crosswise over the thighs and legs so that genital area is easily exposed.

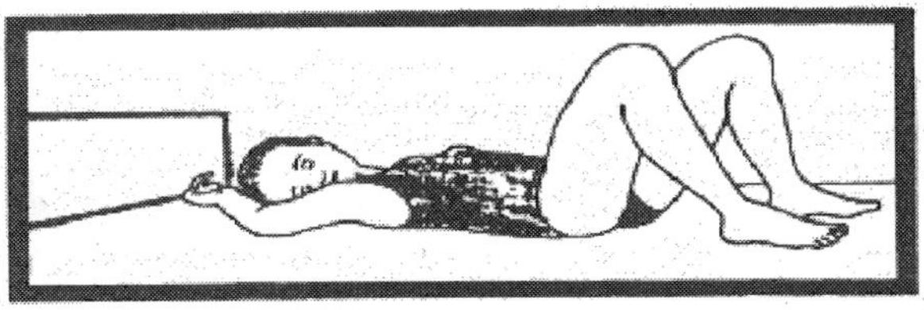

Figure 1-2. Dorsal recumbent position.

c. **Fowler's Position**. Used to promote drainage or ease breathing. Head rest is adjusted to desired height and bed is raised slightly under patient's knees

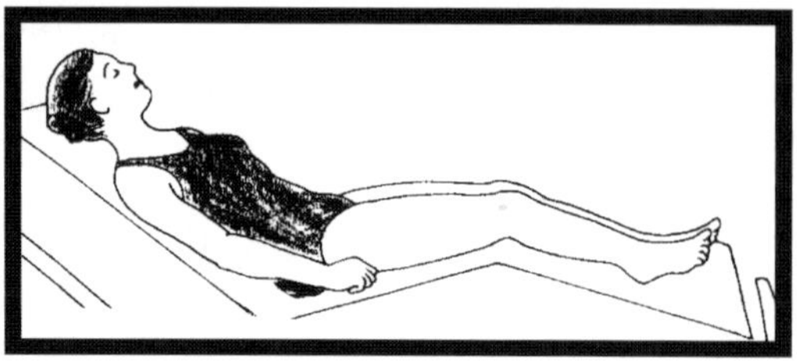

Figure 1-3. Fowler's position.

d. **Dorsal Lithotomy Position**. Used for examination of pelvic organs. Similar to dorsal recumbent position, except that the patient's legs are well separated and thighs are acutely flexed. Feet are usually placed in stirrups. Fold sheet or bath blanket crosswise over thighs and legs so that genital area is easily exposed. Keep patient covered as much as possible.

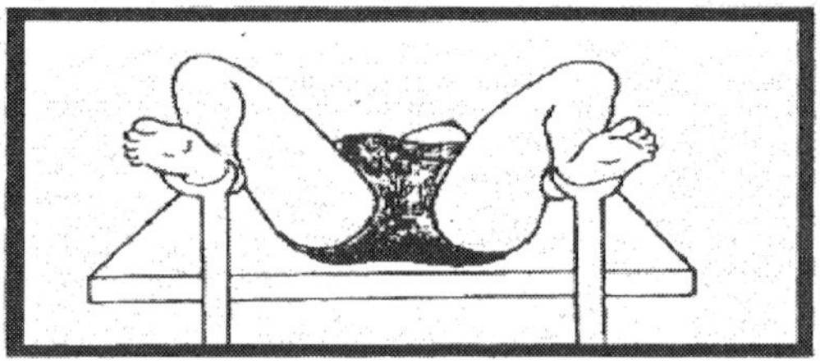

Figure 1-4. Dorsal lithotomy position.

e. **Prone Position**. Used to examine spine and back. Patient lies on abdomen with head turned to one side for comfort. Arms may be above head or alongside body. Cover with sheet or bath blanket.

**NOTE**: An unconscious patient, or one with an abdominal incision or breathing difficulty usually cannot lie in this position.

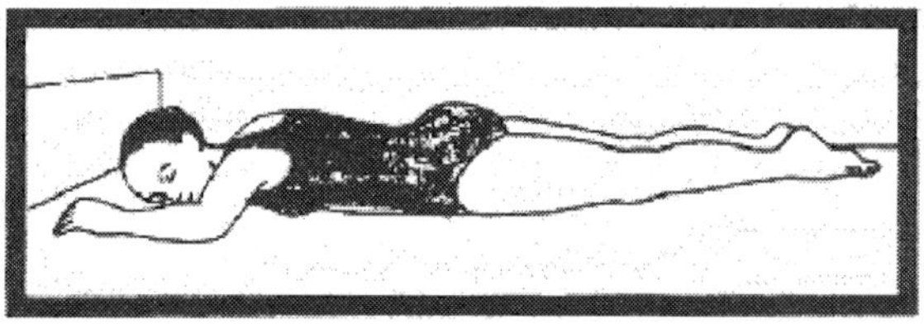

Figure 1-5. Prone position.

f. **Sim's Position.** Used for rectal examination. Patient is on left side with right knee flexed against abdomen and left knee slightly flexed. Left arm is behind body; right arm is placed comfortably.

**NOTE**: Patient with leg injuries or arthritis usually cannot assume this position.

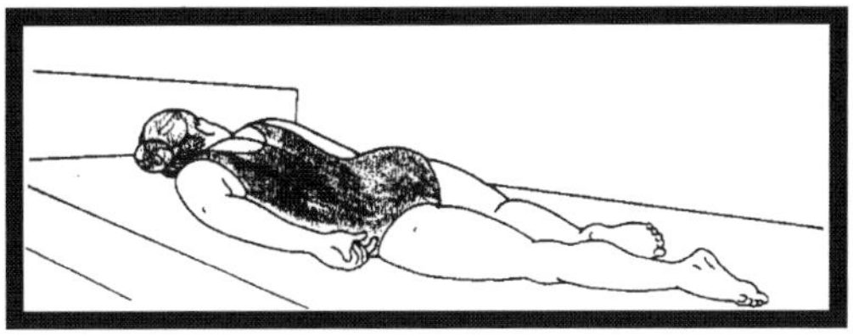

Figure 1-6. Sim's position.

g. **Knee-Chest Position**. Used for rectal and vaginal examinations and as treatment to bring uterus into normal position. Patient is on knees with chest resting on bed and elbows resting on bed or arms above head. Head is turned to one side. Thighs are straight and lower legs are flat on bed.

**NOTE:** Do not leave patient alone; he/she may become dizzy, faint, and fall.

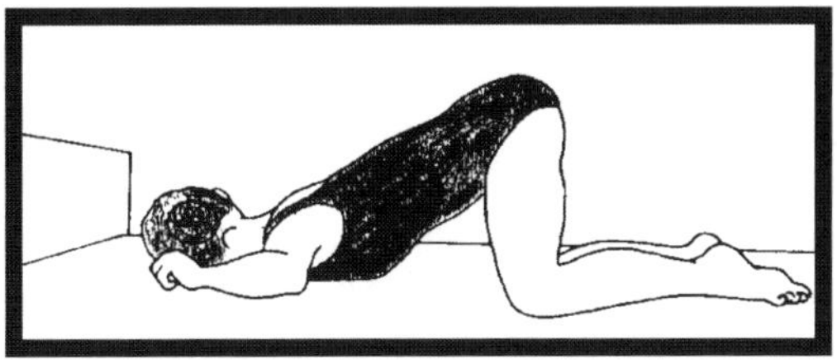

Figure 1-7. Knee-chest position.

## 1-5. BODY SYSTEMS USUALLY EXAMINED BY THE PHYSICIAN

a. **Musculoskeletal System**. The patient should be examined for symmetry of parts, for mobility, and for coordination.

b. **Integumentary System**. The patient's skin should be observed for intactness, color, the presence of scars or rashes, and the skin should be felt for warmth and unusual texture.

c. **Eyes, Ears, Nose, and Throat**. The patient should be examined for patency of passages and cavities, state of balance (equilibrium), and the receptiveness of the sense organs.

d. **Cardiovascular System**. The heart is listened to with a stethoscope to measure the rate, character, and regularity of the heartbeat, as well as to detect any abnormal sounds. Status of the heart and blood vessels is determined by indirectly measuring blood pressure and by directly measuring central venous or arterial pressure. Circulation and pulses in various parts of the body, especially the extremities, may be checked. By looking at blood vessels in the retina with an ophthalmoscope, the physician can infer the condition of the blood vessels in the rest of the body.

e. **Respiratory System**. The respiratory system is evaluated for respiratory rate, adequacy of ventilation and gas exchange membranes, clear lung fields, and symmetry of the chest. The physician can learn a lot about the chest and estimate the size and location of the heart and lungs by auscultation (listening) and by percussion (tapping and thumping). Arterial blood may be drawn to be analyzed for blood gases.

f. **Gastrointestinal (GI) System**. The GI tract is examined for intactness of mucosal membranes, adequacy of digestive process, and regular elimination of solids. Because portions of the digestive tract cannot be seen directly, X-ray procedures, such as a GI series, or gallbladder series are often ordered. Feces may also be examined for the presence of blood or pathogens. The physician may explore the rectum with a gloved finger. The patient is often in the Sims' position for this examination.

g. **Neurologic System**. The neurologic examination evaluates normal reflexes, adequate motor and sensory innervation, development of intellectual and psychological processes. It may consist of assessing the patient's orientation to time and place, assessing sensation by stimulating various parts of the body, and assessing the patient's sense of balance or ability to control body movements. A percussion hammer is used to test reflexes in various parts of the body. In addition, the pupils are checked with a flashlight for reflex. The pupils should quickly contract when a bright light is shined into the eye. The pupils should be round, regular, and of equal size. This is reported as PERRLA (pupils equal, round and reactive to light and accommodation). Accommodation is adjustment, especially of the eye, to variation in distance.

h. **Genitourinary System**. Genitourinary evaluation is to determine adequacy of urinary control and elimination, patency of membranes and passages, and appropriate development of reproductive organs. A vaginal or pelvic examination is done to discover any signs of irritation, growths, displacement, or other abnormal conditions in the pelvic organs or external genitalia. A rectal examination is usually included in the physical examination of a man over 35 years old. This exam aids in discovering cancer of the rectum or prostate gland while it is still in an early stage.

i. **Endocrine System**. The physician may palpate (use hands and fingers to examine) the sex glands and the thyroid gland to determine size and detect any growths. The adequacy of hormonal activity is assessed by observing certain characteristics of body function, growth, and development.

## 1-6. ASSISTING WITH AN INFANT OR CHILD

a. Make every effort to get the child's cooperation during the examination. If the child is too young or too ill to cooperate, use restraint when necessary. Position the child's arms along side the body and wrap the child in a sheet or blanket. Stand on the opposite side of the table from the examiner during the chest and abdominal examination. Hold the child's arms above his head with one of your hands and his feet at the ankles with your other hand.

b. The equipment used to examine an infant or child is the same as for adult except some items are smaller.

## 1-7. PHYSIOLOGICAL MEASUREMENTS ROUTINELY MADE

a. The patient's vital signs (temperature, pulse, respirations), blood pressure, height, and weight should be taken before the examination but 10 to 15 minutes after the patient has rested.

b. Routine examinations such as complete blood count (CBC) with differential, urinalysis, electrolytes, and chest x-ray are usually ordered. Complete the lab and x-ray request slips with the patient's name, rank, social security number, date, and all other required information.

c. Have the results from all lab tests available so that the health care provider can observe/assess and be aware of any abnormal lab values.

## 1-8. PURPOSES FOR DRAPING THE PATIENT DURING THE PHYSICAL EXAM

The patient should be drapped:

a. To prevent unnecessary exposure of the patient's body.

b. To help the patient relax—a patient who is embarrassed will be tense and less cooperative.

c. To prevent chilling — the drapes will provide warmth.

## 1-9. EVALUATION OF A PATIENT'S CONDITION AND NEED FOR ASSISTANCE

Your presence will be comforting for most patients. Some parts of the examination may be uncomfortable or painful. Evaluate the patient's condition and his need for assistance prior to the physical examination. Some factors to consider are:

a. **Age**. Elderly patients will probably need help getting to the examination room, getting on the examination table and assuming certain positions. Infants and children will not be cooperative and may need restraining.

b. **Level of Understanding**. Patients who are confused, unable to understand English, or very young may need nonverbal communication such as a smile or soft pat to assure them. Most patients will not understand medical terms. Assist them by explaining the examination and answering their questions in common language.

c. **Ability to Move**. Disabled patients who move poorly or not at all may need assistance.

d. **State of Health**. Some patients may be just too sick to tolerate a lengthy physical examination. Do not leave very ill or debilitated patients alone; assist them to move and remain in the various positions and observe them for fatigue.

**1-10. CLOSING**

The practical nurse that is assigned to assist in the physical examination plays an important role in supporting both the patient and the physician or other health care providers. Upon completion, chart that the examination was done, by whom, the patient's reaction, and any specimens sent to the lab or special procedures to be followed.

Continue with Exercises

**EXERCISE, LESSON 1**

**INSTRUCTIONS:** To complete this exercise, circle the letter of the response that best answers the question or completes the statement or write the answer in the space provided. After you have completed the all of the exercises, turn to "Solutions to Exercises" at the end of this lesson and check your answers. If you have responded to any of the exercises incorrectly, reread the material referenced after the answer.

1. As a practical nurse who may be called upon to assist the health care provider during a physical examination, you should know the basics of the examination in order to ________________________________________ and so that you may _____________________________________________________.

2. Two purposes for performing the physical examination are
   a. _______________________________________________ and

   b. _______________________________________________.

3. You should have the patient void into a urine specimen cup in order to _____________________________ and to ___________________________.

4. If a male is examining a female, or vice versa, you should __________________ to protect the patient, the health care provider, and the hospital or clinic.

5. You should ____________________________ if the patient has a draining wound, is bleeding, is vomiting, or has an infection.

6. You should _______________________________________ because the physician needs to know the information that has been obtained through the nursing observations and lab reports.

7. To provide continuing privacy for the patient, be sure to __________________ each time the patient assumes a different position during the examination.

8. The health care providers who could perform the physical examination are the ______________, __________________ or ________________________.

9. Four body systems that the health care provider would usually examine during a physical examination are:

   a. ____________________________________________.

   b. ____________________________________________.

   c. ____________________________________________.

   d. ____________________________________________.

10. When restraining a child during the physical examination, you should:

    a. Hold the child's arms above his head with one hand and hold his feet at the ankles with your other hand.

    b. Stand on the opposite side of the table from the examiner.

    c. Place the child's arms alongside his body and wrap him in a sheet or blanket.

    d. All of the above.

11. Physiological measurements, which are routinely made, are the patient's __________, ______________________, ______________________, and ______________________________ and lab test such as ______________________________, _________________________, and ______________________________.

12. The purposes for draping the patient during physical examination are to ______________________________, to ______________________________, and to ______________________________.

13. Factors that indicate the patient's need for assistance are __________________, ______________________________, ______________________________, and ______________________________.

***Check Your Answers on Next Page***

## SOLUTIONS TO EXERCISE, LESSON 1

1. Have the appropriate equipment and supplies on hand;
   place the patient in the proper position and drape him correctly. (para 1-1)

2. Any **two** of these are correct:
   To determine the patient's level of health or psychological function.
   To arrive at a tentative diagnosis.
   To confirm a diagnosis.
   To evaluate the effectiveness of prescribed medical treatment and therapy.
   (paras 1-2a--d)

3. Empty the bladder;
   obtain a urine specimen for urinalysis. (para 1-3b)

4. Stay in the room. (para 1-3d)

5. Wear gloves. (para 1-3e)

6. Have the patient's chart available. (para 1-3f)

7. Adjust the drapes. (para 1-3h)

8. Physician, nurse practitioner, physician assistant. (para 1-2)

9. Any **four** of the following are correct:
   Musculoskeletal.
   Integumentary.
   Eyes, ears, nose, and throat.
   Cardiovascular.
   Respiratory.
   Gastrointestinal.
   Neurologic.
   Genitourinary.
   Endocrine. (paras 1-5a--i)

10. d (para 1-6a)

11. Vital signs, blood pressure, height, and weight;
    CBC with differential, urinalysis, and electrolytes. (paras 1-7a--b)

12. Prevent unnecessary exposure, help the patient relax, prevent chilling.
    (paras 1-8a--c)

13. Age; level of understanding; ability to move; state of health. (paras 1-9a--d)

End of Lesson 1

## LESSON ASSIGNMENT

**LESSON 2** Specimen Collection

**TEXT ASSIGNMENT** Paragraphs 2-1 through 2-19

**LESSON OBJECTIVES** After completing this lesson, you should be able to:

2-1. Select the principles, supplies and equipment, and procedures, which apply to obtaining a sample for throat culture.

2-2. Select the principles, supplies and equipment, and procedures, which apply to obtaining a sputum specimen.

2-3. Select the principles, supplies and equipment, and procedures that apply to obtaining a stool specimen.

2-4. Identify the steps of the procedure for correctly obtaining a midstream urine specimen, a 24-hour urine collection, and urine for a pregnancy test.

2-5. Identify abnormalities in the color and odor of urine.

2-6. Select the reason for obtaining a blood culture.

**SUGGESTION** After studying the assignment, complete the exercises at the end of this lesson. These exercises will help you to achieve the lesson objectives.

# LESSON 2

# SPECIMEN COLLECTION

## 2-1. INTRODUCTION

One means of gathering information about the patient's health status is by identifying pathogens and analyzing urine, blood, sputum, and feces. As a practical nurse, you may be responsible for collecting and labeling specimen for analysis and ensuring their delivery to the lab. For self-protection and to prevent the spread of disease, wear gloves whenever you work with body fluids. Washing your hands carefully also prevents the spread of disease.

## 2-2. THROAT CULTURE

Throat cultures are done to isolate and identify any pathogens, which may be medium. The slide or medium is incubated in the laboratory to determine which organisms causing a throat disorder. A sample of mucus and secretions from the back of the throat is collected on a cotton-tipped applicator and applied to a slide or culture are present. A determination of which drug is most effective against a particular organism may be done also. A full culture and sensitivity test takes several days because the organisms must have time to grow. If strep infection is suspected a quick strep test may be done, so that antibiotic therapy can be started immediately.

## 2-3. SUPPLIES AND EQUIPMENT

The supplies and equipment required to obtain a sample for throat culture are:

a. Sterile cotton-tipped applicator specimen collection kit (culturette).

b. Tongue depressor.

c. Laboratory request form.

d. Flashlight.

## 2-4. PROCEDURE FOR A THROAT CULTURE

Always wash your hands before the procedure. Explain to the patient what you are going to do. Have the patient sit comfortably on a bed or chair and tilt his head back.

a. Use the flashlight to illuminate the back of the throat. Check for inflamed areas using the tongue depressor.

b. Ask the patient to say "Ahhh" as you swab the tonsillar areas from side to side. Be sure to include any inflamed of purulent sites.

c. Avoid touching the tongue, cheeks, or teeth with the applicator, as this will contaminate it with oral bacteria.

d. Place the cotton-tipped applicator into the culture tube immediately.

e. Label the culture tube with the patient's name, SSN, and ward number if applicable.

f. Complete the request form (SF 553) with the following information:

(1) Patient's name.

(2) Patient's rank or status.

(3) Family member prefix and sponsor's social security number.

(4) Ward number if inpatient, or phone number if outpatient.

(5) Source of the specimen (that is, throat).

(6) Any antibiotics the patient is taking.

(7) Date and time the specimen was obtained.

(8) Name of the physician who ordered the culture.

## 2-5. SPUTUM SPECIMEN

For some respiratory disorders, a sputum specimen is obtained for culture or other examination to determine if any pathogens or blood are present. The specimen should be collected early in the morning before the patient eats, brushes his teeth, or uses mouthwash. The specimen is more likely to contain sputum at this time, rather than just saliva. Specimens are often taken for three consecutive days because it is difficult for the patient to cough up enough sputum at one time, and an organism may be missed if only one culture is done.

## 2-6. SUPPLIES AND EQUIPMENT

Supplies and equipment required to collect a sputum specimen are

a. Sterile container with tight-fitting lid.

b. Box of tissues.

c. Gloves.

d. Laboratory request form (SF 553).

## 2-7. PROCEDURE FOR SPUTUM SPECIMEN

a. Wash your hands and gather the equipment.

b. Provide privacy for the patient and explain the procedure. Place the tissues nearby and have the patient rinse his mouth with clear water to remove any food particles.

c. Assist the patient to a sitting position, if necessary and ask him to cough deeply and spit into the container. Tell the patient to avoid touching the inside of the container because it is sterile.

d. A sputum specimen is considered highly contaminated and must be treated with caution. To prevent contamination by particles in the air, keep the container closed until the patient is ready to spit into it. Close the container immediately after collecting the specimen to prevent the spread of any organisms from the specimen. Offer tissues for the patient to wipe his mouth.

e. Wash your hands, label the container, and complete the laboratory request form. Take the specimen to the laboratory immediately; allowing the specimen to remain in a warm place will result in overgrowth of any organisms that may be present.

f. Record the amount, consistency, and color of the sputum collected, as well as the time and date in the nursing notes.

## 2-8. STOOL SPECIMEN

Stool specimen are collected for many examinations. The most common is the ova and parasites test, a microscopic examination of feces for detecting parasites such as amebas or worms. Stools specimen are often tested for blood. Guaiac or HemOccult test may be done in the laboratory but are sometimes done at the nursing station to test a stool for occult blood.

## 2-9. SUPPLIES AND EQUIPMENT

Supplies and equipment required to collect a stool specimen are

a. Gloves

b. Clean bedpan and cover (an extra bedpan or urinal if the patient must void).

c. Specimen container and lid.

d. Wooden tongue blades.

e. Paper bag for used tongue blades.

e. Labels.

f. Plastic bag for transport of container with specimen to laboratory.

## 2-10. PROCEDURE FOR STOOL SPECIMEN

a. Explain the reason for the test and the procedure to the patient. Ask the patient to tell you when he feels the urge to have a bowel movement.

b. Wear gloves when handling any bodily discharge (see standard precautions in the introduction to this subcourse).

c. Give the bedpan when the patient is ready. If the patient wants to urinate first, give a male the urinal or give a female the extra bedpan.

d. Remove the bedpan. Use the tongue blade to transfer a portion of the feces to the specimen container. Do not touch the specimen because it is contaminated. It is not necessary to keep this specimen sterile however, because the gastrointestinal tract is not sterile.

e. Cover the container and label it with the patient's name and social security number.

f. Complete the appropriate laboratory request form, noting any special examination ordered.

g. Take the specimen to the lab immediately; examination for parasites, ova, and organisms must be made while the stool is warm.

h. If an infant's stool is to be examined, place the diaper in a leakproof bag, label it, and take the diaper and request form to the lab immediately.

## 2-11. GUAIAC TEST

The purpose of this test, using guaiac as a reagent, is to detect the presence of occult blood (blood that appears from a nonspecific source, with obscure signs and symptoms), which is not visible. Each method of testing has a specific procedure, which must be followed to get accurate results. If it is done at the nursing station, instructions should be kept with the reagents used. Follow the manufacturer's instructions or consult hospital standing operating procedures (SOP).

## 2-12. URINE SPECIMENS

Urinalysis is included in a health examination, and as part of the admission process for all inpatients. Simple urine tests, such as for sugar and acetone, are often performed by the nurse in the hospital or by the patient at home. Urine is assessed first for its physical appearance:

a. **Color**. Freshly voided urine is transparent and light amber in color. The amount and kinds of waste in the urine make it lighter or darker. Blood in the urine colors it; if the amount of blood in the urine is great, the urine will be red. During a flare-up of chronic nephritis, the small number of red blood cells present in the urine give it a smoky appearance.

b. **Odor**. Freshly voided urine has a characteristic odor. When urine stands, decomposition from bacterial activity gives it an ammonia-like odor. Refrigerate the urine sample if it is not to be examined at once.

## 2-13. MIDSTREAM URINE SPECIMEN

Midstream (clean-catch) urine collection is the most common method of obtaining urine specimens from adults, particularly men. This method allows a specimen, which is not contaminated from external sources to be obtained without catheterization.

a. **Supplies and Equipment**.

(1) Sterile specimen cup.

(2) Zephiran, a soap solution, or three antiseptic towelettes.

(3) Three cotton balls (to use with zephiran or soap solution).

(4) Laboratory request form.

b. **Procedure**.

(1) Instruct the patient to clean the urethral area thoroughly. This will prevent external bacteria from entering the specimen. The female should wipe from front to back to avoid contaminating the vaginal and urethral area from the anal area. She should clean each side with a separate cotton ball or towelette, then use the last one for the urethral area itself. The male should cleanse the penis, using the first cotton ball or towelette for the urethral meatus, the next cotton ball to clean the end of the penis, and the last to cleanse the urethral opening.

(2) Instruct the patient to void a small amount of urine into the toilet to rinse out the urethra, void the midstream urine into the specimen cup, and the last of the stream into the toilet. The midstream urine is considered to be bladder and kidney washings; the portion that the physician wants tested.

(3) Complete the laboratory request form, label the specimen container with patient identifying information, and send to the lab immediately. A delay in examining the specimen may cause a false result when bacterial determinations are to be made.

(4) Wash your hands and instruct the patient to do likewise.

(5) Record that the specimen was collected. Note any difficulties the patient had or if the urine had an abnormal appearance.

## 2-14. 24-HOUR URINE SPECIMEN

A 24-hour urine collection always begins with an empty bladder so that the urine collected is not "left over" from previous hours. This specimen shows the total amounts of wastes the kidneys are eliminating and the amount of each.

a. **Supplies and Equipment.**

(1) Large, clean bottle with cap or stopper.

(2) Measuring graduate.

(3) Bedpan or urinal.

(4) Refrigerated storage area.

(5) Gloves.

b. **Procedure**.

(1) Label the bottle with patient identifying information, the date, and time the collection begins and ends.

(2) Instruct the patient to void all urine into a bedpan or urinal. Measure each specimen of urine voided and pour into the refrigerated bottle. Wash your hands before and after each collection. Record each amount on the intake and output (I&O) sheet.

(3) Exactly 24-hours after beginning the collection, ask the patient to void. This will complete the specimen collection.

(4) Send the bottle and laboratory request form to the lab.

## 2-15. PREGNANCY URINE TEST

Most pregnancy tests are based on the fact that the hormone human chorionic gonadotropin (HCG) is secreted by the chorionic villi of the placenta. This hormone can be detected in small amounts in both the urine and the blood of a pregnant woman by the 15th day of pregnancy. Urine tests are available for home use and offer quick results with 90 percent to 95 percent accuracy.

a. **Supplies and Equipment**. Only a urine specimen cup is required.

b. **Procedure**.

(1) Instruct the patient to void the very first urine when she gets up in the morning into the specimen cup.

(2) Label the specimen cup with the patient's identifying information, complete a laboratory request form (Chemistry I, SF 546) requesting an HCG test and send both to the lab.

(3) Only the physician or a registered nurse should tell the patient the results of the test.

## 2-16. BLOOD CULTURES

Blood cultures are done to identify a disease-causing organism, especially in patients who have an elevated temperature for an unknown reason. Drawing blood from HIV positive patients is done in accordance with the hospital or clinic's local policy (see standardl precautions).

## 2-17. SUPPLIES AND EQUIPMENT

Supplies and equipment required for a blood culture are

a. Sterile syringe (20 cc) and three needles (usually 20 gauge).

b. Two blood culture bottles (one for anaerobic and one for aerobic specimens).

c. Betadine solution.

d. Sterile cotton balls or gauze pads.

e. Gloves.

f. Tourniquet.

g. Band-aid®.

h. Chux® (to protect the bed)

i. Laboratory request form.

## 2-18. PROCEDURE FOR BLOOD CULTURES

a. Explain the procedure and the reason for doing the procedure to the patient.

b. Gather all supplies and equipment and bring to the patient's bedside.

c. Assist the patient to a comfortable position. If the patient is uncooperative or disoriented, get someone to help you.

d. Carefully wash your hands.

e. Clean the top of both culture bottles with betadine solution.

f. Put the needle on the syringe.

g. Apply the tourniquet.

h. Put on the gloves and clean the drawing site with betadine solution.

i. Draw at least 10 cc of blood from the patient (5 cc is needed for each bottle).

j. Loosen the tourniquet.

k. Remove the syringe and needle while applying pressure to the venipuncture site with the cotton ball or gauze pad. Have the patient apply pressure to the site.

l. Replace the needle on the syringe with another sterile needle.

m. Inject 5 cc of blood into the anaerobic bottle; do not allow air to enter the bottle.

n. Replace the needle on the syringe with another sterile needle.

o. Inject 5 cc of blood into the aerobic bottle and while the needle is still in the bottle, disconnect it from the syringe so that air enters the aerobic bottle.

p. Gently mix the blood with the solution in both bottles.

q. Label both bottles with patient identifying information and the type of culture hat is, aerobic or anaerobic).

r. Complete laboratory request forms and send the specimens to the laboratory immediately.

s. Place a band-aid over the patient's venipuncture site.

## 2-19. CLOSING

The role you play in collecting and labeling specimens and ensuring their timely delivery to the lab for analysis is a very important one. Carefully follow the steps of each procedure to prevent contaminating the specimen or spreading infection. Always document that the procedure was done and by whom.

Continue with Exercises

**EXERCISE, LESSON 2**

**INSTRUCTIONS:** To complete this exercise, circle the letter of the response that best answers the question or completes the statement or write the answer in the space provided. After you have completed the all of the exercises, turn to "Solutions to Exercises" at the end of this lesson and check your answers. If you have responded to any of the exercises incorrectly, reread the material referenced after the answer.

1. For self-protection and to prevent the spread of disease, you should ______________________________ and ______________________________ when collecting specimens for laboratory analysis.

2. A throat culture is done to ______________________________ ______________________________ that may be causing a throat disorder.

3. A full culture and sensitivity test takes ______________________________.

4. The supplies and equipment required to obtain a sample for throat culture are:

   a. ______________________________.

   b. ______________________________.

   c. ______________________________.

   d. ______________________________.

5. Which of the following is <u>not</u> a correct step in collecting a sample for throat culture.

   a. Illuminate the back of the throat.

   b. Swab inflamed and purulent sites in the tonsillar area.

   c. Swab the tongue and cheeks before placing the cotton-tipped applicator into the culture tube.

   d. Label the culture tube with the patient's name, SSAN, and ward number.

6. A sputum specimen should be collected________________________________.

7. Supplies and equipment required to collect a sputum specimen are:

   a. ____________________________________________.

   b. ____________________________________________.

   c. ____________________________________________.

   d. ____________________________________________.

8. A sputum specimen is treated with caution because it is considered
   ________________________________

9. The most common examination for which a stool specimen is collected is the
   _____________________________________.

10. The hormone HCG can be detected in the urine and blood of a
    __________________________.

11. After collecting a sputum specimen, you should record in the Nurses Notes:

    a. ____________________________________________.

    b. ____________________________________________.

    c. ____________________________________________.

    d. ____________________________________________.

12. _______________ or ______________________ may be done at the nursing station to test a stool specimen for occult blood.

13. Urine should be assessed first for its physical appearance. Freshly voided urine is __________________ and ____________________ in color.

14. When urine stands, decomposition from bacterial activity gives it an ___________________________ odor.

15. The most common method of obtaining urine from adults is ________________________________ collection.

16. Supplies and equipment required for a clean-catch urine collection are:

    a. ______________________________________________.

    b. ______________________________________________.

    c. ______________________________________________.

    d. ______________________________________________.

17. A _______________________ urine collection always begins with an empty bladder so that none of the urine collected is "left over" from previous hours.

18. A large, clean bottle and refrigerated storage area is used for a _________________________urine collection.

19. A ___________________ is done to identify a disease-causing organism, especially in patients who have an elevated temperature for an unknown reason.

20. A sterile 20 cc syringe, three sterile 20 gauge needles, betadine solution, a tourniquet and a Band-aid® are required to collect a specimen for ___________________________________________.

Check Your Answers on Next Page

## SOLUTIONS TO EXERCISE, LESSON 2

1. Wear gloves; wash hands carefully. (para 2-1)

2. Isolate and identify any pathogens that may be causing a throat disorder. (para 2-2)

3. Several days. (para 2-2)

4. The following in any order.
   Sterile cotton-tipped applicator or culturette.
   Tongue depressor.
   Laboratory request form.
   Flashlight. (paras 2-3a--d)

5. c (para 2-4a-e)

6. Early in the morning. (para 2-5)

7. The following in any order.
   Sterile container with tight fitting lid.
   Box of tissues.
   Gloves.
   Lab request form (SF 553). (paras 2-6a--d)

8. Highly contaminated. (para 2-7d)

9. Ova and parasites test. (para 2-8)

10. Pregnant woman. (para 2-15)

11. The following in any order.
    The amount of sputum.
    Consistency of sputum.
    Color of sputum.
    Time and date collected. (para 2-7f)

12. Guaiac; HemOccult test. (para 2-8)

13. Transparent; light amber. (para 2-12a)

14. Ammonia-like. (para 2-12b)

15. Midstream (clean-catch). (para 2-13)

16. The following in any order.
    Sterile specimen cup.
    Zephiran, a soap solution, or antiseptic towelettes.
    Cotton balls.
    Lab request form. (para-2-13a(1)--(4))

17. 24-hour. (para 2-14)

18. 24-hour. (para 2-14a)

19. Blood culture. (para 2-16)

20. Blood culture. (paras 2-17a-i)

End of Lesson 2

## LESSON ASSIGNMENT

**LESSON 3** Catheterization of the Male and Female Patient

**TEXT ASSIGNMENT** Paragraphs 3-1 through 3-11

**LESSON OBJECTIVES** After completing this lesson, you should be able to:

3-1. Select the purposes of urinary catheterization.

3-2. Identify three types of urinary catheters.

3-3. Select nursing implications, which apply to care of a patient with an indwelling urinary catheter.

3-4. Select the appropriate equipment and technique used in catheterizing a male patient.

3-5. Select the appropriate equipment and technique used in catheterizing a female patient.

3-6. Select the appropriate equipment and technique used to remove a Foley catheter.

**SUGGESTION** After studying the assignment, complete the exercises at the end of this lesson. These exercises will help you to achieve the lesson objectives.

# LESSON 3

## CATHETERIZATION OF THE MALE AND FEMALE PATIENT

### 3-1. INTRODUCTION

Catheterization of the urinary bladder is the insertion of a hollow tube through the urethra into the bladder for removing urine. It is an aseptic procedure for which sterile equipment is required.

### 3-2. PURPOSES OF URINARY CATHETERIZATION

Purposes for urinary catheterization include the following.

a. **Relieve Urinary Retention**. Urine retained in the bladder for any reason causes the patient discomfort and increases the likelihood of infection. A catheter may be inserted to relieve urinary retention when a patient is temporarily unable to void or has difficulty releasing urine from the bladder due to an obstruction of the urethra or at the meatus.

b. **Obtain a Sterile Urine Specimen from a Female Patient**. At one time, this was considered necessary to obtain a urine specimen entirely free of contamination. Most physicians now order a collection of a voided, midstream clean-catch specimen.

c. **Measure Residual Urine**. Catheterization can be done to measure the amount of residual urine in the bladder when voiding only partly empties it.

d. **Empty the Bladder Before, During, or After Surgery**. A catheter may be inserted before or following abdominal surgery, especially if the patient cannot be up and about. Catheterization to keep the bladder empty of urine during a surgical procedure permits the surgeon a better view and palpation of internal tissue, and prevents accidental injury to the bladder. Catheterization may also be used to prevent urine from touching sutures in the perineum.

### 3-3. URINARY CATHETER SIZES

The French scale (Fr.) is used to denote the size of catheters. Each unit is roughly equivalent to 0.33 mm in diameter (that is, 18 Fr. indicates a diameter of 6 mm). The smaller the number, the smaller the catheter. A larger sized catheter is used for a male because it is stiffer, thus easier to push the distance of the male urethra. Catheters come in several sizes:

a. Number 8 Fr. and 10 Fr. are used for children.

b. Number 14 Fr. and 16 Fr. are used for female adults.

c. Number 20 Fr. and 22 Fr. are usually used for male adults.

## 3-4. TYPES OF URINARY CATHETERS

The catheters most commonly used are made of plastic. Each type of catheter (figure 3-1) has a rounded tip to prevent injury to the meatus or the urethra. The Foley catheter is frequently used. It is usually inserted by the nurse. The Malecot four-wing catheter and the dePezzer mushroom catheter are inserted by the urologist using a stylet. The stylet is removed after the catheter has been inserted. Because they are very difficult to sterilize, catheters should be considered disposable and discarded after they have been removed.

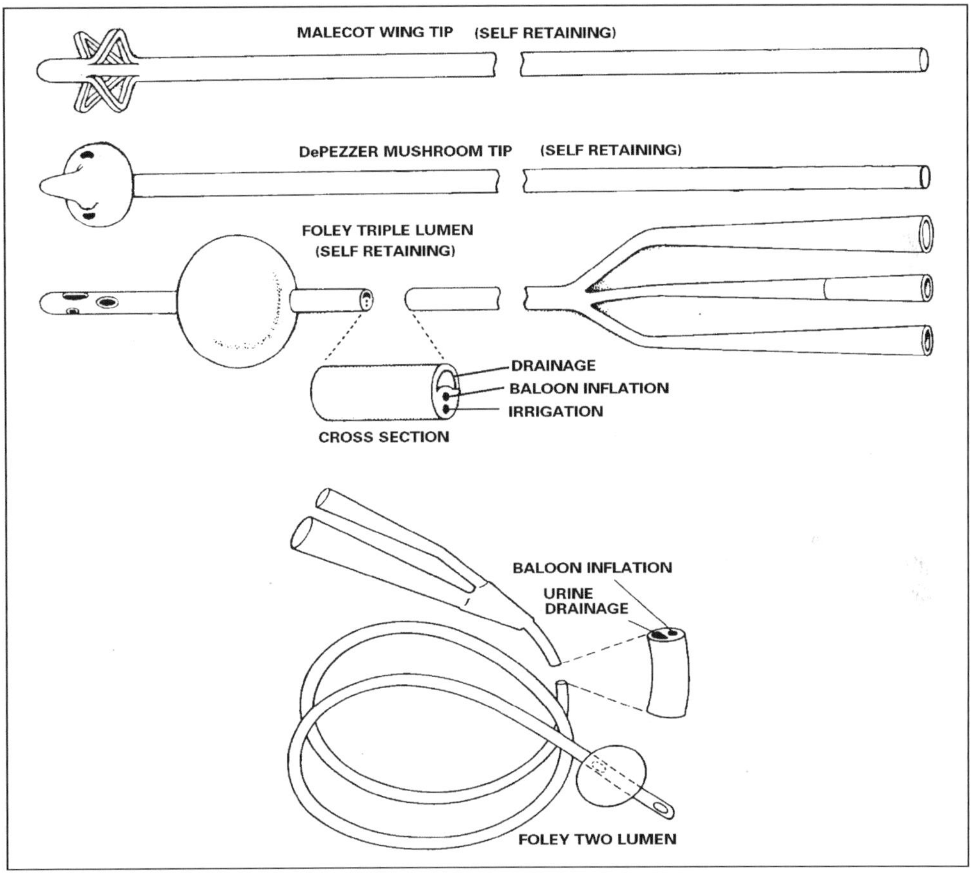


Figure 3-1. Urinary catheters.

a. **Intermittent Catheter**. An intermittent catheter is used to drain the bladder for short periods (5-10 minutes). It may be inserted by the patient.

b. **Retention/Indwelling Catheter**. This type of catheter is placed into the bladder and secured there for a period of time. It is used following surgery, bladder injury, or in bladder infections. It may also be used for an incontinent or nonresponsive patient.

(1) It provides continuous temporary or permanent drainage of urine.

(2) It is used for gradual decompression of an over distended bladder.

(3) It is used for intermittent drainage and irrigation.

(4) The most commonly used indwelling catheter is the Foley catheter. A drainage tube and collection device are connected to the catheter. It has a balloon at the distal end, which is inflated with sterile water or saline to prevent the catheter from slipping out of the bladder. It is multi-lumened (having several passages within the catheter). One lumen provides a passage for fluid to inflate the balloon. This passage may be self-sealing or may require a clamp. The second lumen is the passage through which the urine drains. Some indwelling catheters have a third lumen for instilling irrigation fluid.

c. **Supra Pubic Catheter**. This type of catheter is inserted into the bladder through a small incision above the pubic area. It is used for continuous drainage.

## 3-5. PREPARING FOR CATHETERIZATION

A catheter should be used only when absolutely necessary and the catheterization procedure itself should be done only by trained personnel under sterile conditions. Infection is a major risk of urinary catheterization.

a. **Gather All Equipment**.

(1) Disposable indwelling catheter kit. The kit contains the required equipment needed for catheterization and is packaged to ensure that the equipment is sterile. The kit includes the catheter, a drape, a receptacle to receive urine, materials to clean the area of insertion, a lubricant, a specimen container, and sterile gloves.

(2) Flashlight or lamp.

(3) Urine collection bag.

(4) Velcro leg strap or anchoring tape.

(5) Disposal bag.

(6) Waterproof pad or Chux®.

b. **Explain the Procedure to the Patient**. Advise the patient that he may feel a burning sensation and pressure as the catheter is inserted, and that he will feel that he needs to void after the catheter is in place. Do not suggest to the patient that he may feel pain; however, introducing a catheter in swollen or injured tissue may cause discomfort.

c. **Provide for Privacy and Adequate Lighting**.

(1) Close the door or pull the curtain surrounding the patient's bed and position the flashlight or lamp at the end of the bed.

(2) Position the female patient in a dorsal recumbent position with the knees flexed and the feet about two feet apart. Place Chux® under the patient's buttocks. Cover the upper body and each leg. Place the catheter set between the female patient's legs.

(3) Position a male patient in a supine position. Place Chux® under the patient's buttocks. Drape the patient so that only the area around the penis is exposed. Place the catheter set next to the legs of the male patient.

## 3-6. INSERTING THE FOLEY CATHETER IN A MALE PATIENT

The following procedures are used to insert the Foley catheter in a male patient.

a. Cleanse the genital and perineal areas with warm soap and water. Rinse and dry.

b. Wash your hands carefully.

c. Open the sterile catheterization kit, using sterile technique.

d. Put on the sterile gloves.

e. Open the sterile drape and place on the patient's thighs. Place fenestrated drape with opening on the penis.

f. Apply sterile lubricant liberally to the catheter tip. Lubricate at least six inches of the catheter. Leave the lubricated catheter on the sterile field.

g. Pour the antiseptic solution over the cotton balls.

h. Place the urine specimen collection container within easy reach.

i. Grasp the patient's penis between your thumb and forefinger of your nondominant hand. Retract the foreskin of an uncircumcised male. The gloved hand that has touched the patient is now contaminated.

j. Use the forceps to hold the cotton balls (figure 3-2). This will maintain the sterility of one hand. Using the forceps, pick up one cotton ball and swab the center of the meatus outward in a circular manner.

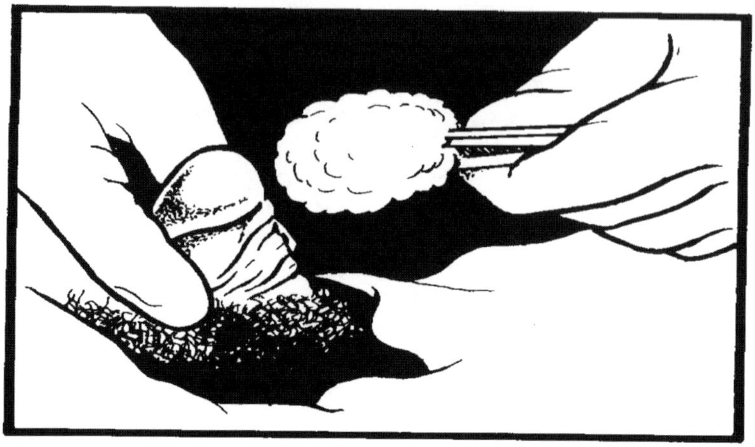

Figure 3-2. Cleansing the male meatus.

k. Continue outward, using a new cotton ball for each progressively larger circle. Clean the entire glands. Deposit each cotton ball in the disposal bag. After the last cotton ball is used, drop the forceps into the disposal bag as well.

l. Hold the penis at a 90-degree angle (figure 3-3). Advance the catheter into the patient's urinary meatus. You may encounter resistance at the prostatic sphincter.

(1) Pause and allow the sphincter to relax.

(2) Lower the penis and continue to advance the catheter.

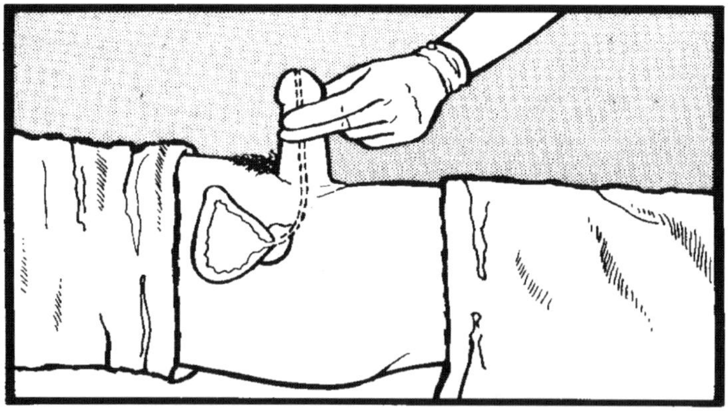

Figure 3-3. Positioning the penis at a 90-degree angle

**NOTE:** Never force the catheter to advance. Discontinue the procedure if the catheter will not advance or the patient has unusual discomfort. Get assistance from the charge nurse or physician.

m. When the catheter has passed through the prostatic sphincter into the bladder, urine will start to flow into the collection bag if it is preconnected. If it is not preconnected, collect a specimen if required, then place the end of the catheter into the tubing of the sterile receptacle.

n. Attach the syringe to the balloon port and inject the water slowly to inflate the balloon. Connect the urine collection bag if it is not preconnected.

o. Anchor the catheter tubing to the lateral abdomen with tape (figure 3-4).

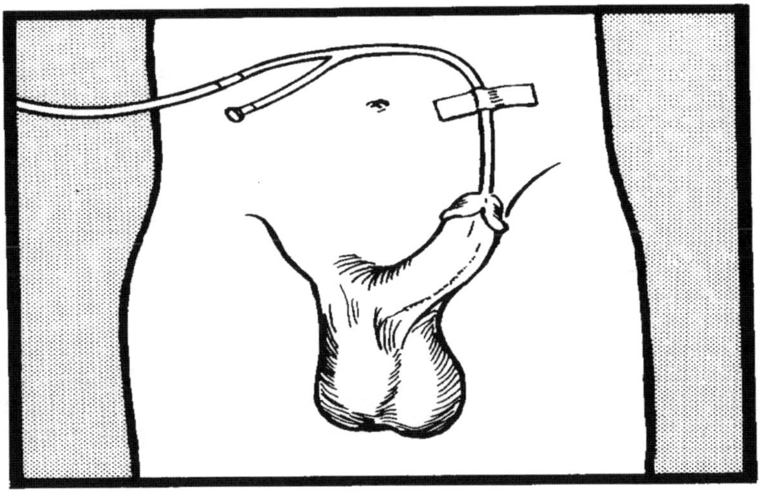

Figure 3-4. Anchoring (male) indwelling catheter.

p. Secure the urinary collection bag below the level of the bladder and off the floor. Coil any extra tubing on the bed.

q. Remove your gloves, the drapes and protectors from around the patient, and any lubricant or antiseptic on the patient's skin.

r. Discard disposable equipment and return reusable equipment to the appropriate area.

s. Record the time that the procedure was done and by whom, the patient's reaction to the procedure, all patient teaching done and the patient's level of understanding. Report any significant observations to the charge nurse to include:

(1) The amount, color, and clarity of the urine.

(2) Any difficulties with the procedure.

(3) The presence of blood in the urine.

## 3-7. INSERTING THE FOLEY CATHETER IN A FEMALE PATIENT

The following procedures are used to insert the Foley catheter in a female patient.

a. Wash the area around the meatus with warm soap and water. Rinse and dry.

b. Wash your hands.

c. Open the sterile catheterization kit, using sterile technique.

d. Put on sterile gloves.

e. Place the fenestrated drape on the patient with the hole over the female genitalia.

f. Apply sterile lubricant liberally to the catheter tip. Lubricate at least three inches of the catheter for the female. Leave the lubricated catheter over the cotton balls.

g. Place the urine specimen collection container within reach.

h. Place the thumb and forefinger of your nondominant hand between the labia minora, spread and separate upward. The gloved hand that has touched the patient is now contaminated.

i. Using the forceps, pick up a cotton ball saturated with antiseptic solution. Use one cotton ball for each stroke. Swab from above the meatus downward toward the rectum.

j. Keeping the labia separated, cleanse each side of the meatus in the same downward manner (figure 3-5). Do not go back over any previously cleansed area.

k. Deposit each cotton ball into the disposal bag. After the last cotton ball is used, deposit the forceps into the bag as well.

l. Continue to hold the labium apart after cleansing. Insert the lubricated catheter into the female patient's urinary meatus (figure 3-6).

m. Angle the catheter upward as it is advanced. If the catheter will not advance, instruct the patient to inhale and exhale slowly. This may relax the sphincter muscle. Do not force the catheter.

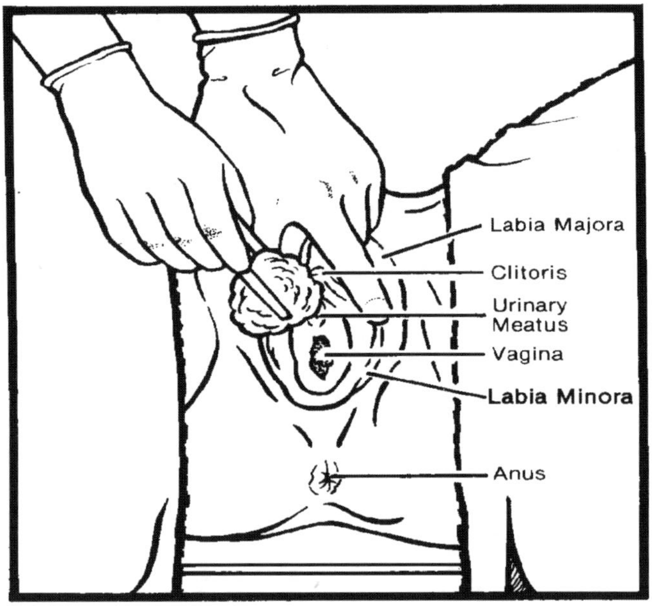


Figure 3-5. Cleansing the female meatus.

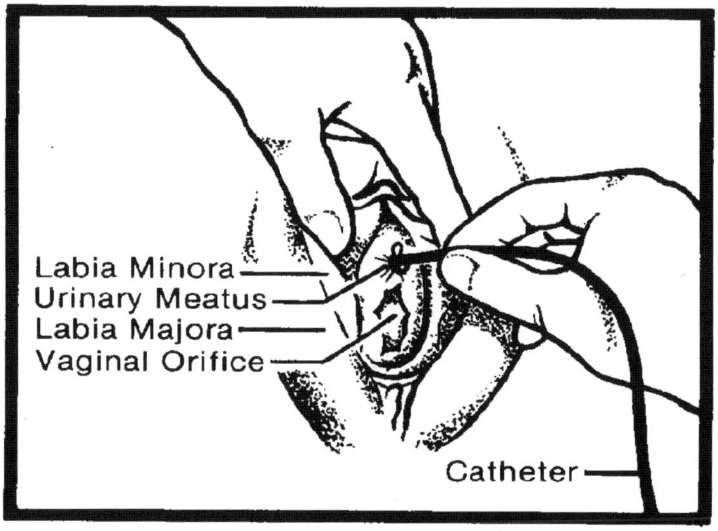


Figure 3-6. Inserting the catheter in a female.

n. When urine starts to flow, insert the catheter approximately one inch further. Place the cup under the stream of flowing urine to obtain a sterile specimen if required.

o. Hold the catheter in place while the urine drains into the collection container.

**NOTE:** If the catheter is inadvertently placed in the patient's vagina, leave it in place temporarily. Insert another catheter properly by repeating the entire procedure using another sterile set; then remove the catheter from the vagina.

p. Attach the syringe to the balloon port of the catheter. Inject the water slowly to inflate the balloon. If the water will not inject easily or the patient complains of pain, deflate the balloon completely and advance the catheter further, then re-inflate.

q. Remove the syringe. To position the balloon correctly, pull on the catheter gently until you feel resistance.

r. Connect the drainage bag to the catheter. Secure the catheter to the inner aspect of the female patient's thigh (figure 3-7).

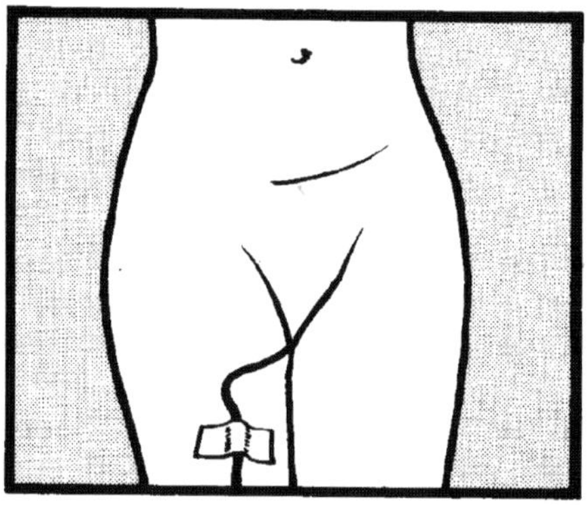

Figure 3-7. Securing (female) indwelling catheter.

s. Attach the urinary drainage bag to the bed, below the level of the bladder but off the floor. Coil any extra tubing on the bed.

t. Remove any lubricant or antiseptic on the patient's skin. Remove your gloves, the drapes and the Chux® from around the patient.

u. Discard disposable equipment and return reusable equipment to the appropriate area.

v. Record the time that the procedure was done and by whom, the patient's reaction to the procedure, all patient teaching done, and the patient's level of understanding. Report observations to the charge nurse to include:

(1) The amount, color, and clarity of the urine.

(2) Any difficulty with the procedure.

(3) The presence of blood in the urine.

## 3-8. MAINTAINING AN INDWELLING CATHETER

When an indwelling or retention catheter is inserted, the nurse is responsible for the daily care required to maintain proper drainage and reduce the possibility of an infection occurring. Always have a confident, reassuring, and professional attitude when maintaining the catheter so that the patient will not feel embarrassed.

a. Wash your hands before and after caring for the patient and wear gloves when handling an indwelling catheter.

b. Clean the perineal area with soap and water twice daily and after each bowel movement, especially around the meatus. Use a separate area of the cloth for each stroke.

c. In some cases, an antiseptic may be used for perineal care. Povidone iodine (Betadine) is most commonly recommended.

d. Avoid use of lotions or powder in the perineal area.

e. Arrange for the patient to take a shower or tub bath when permitted. The collecting container may be hung over the side of the tub. The catheter should be clamped temporarily if the collecting container is higher than the bladder.

f. A leg bag (figure 3-8) may be worn in the shower. This device allows the ambulatory patient to move about freely and dress in his usual clothing. Keep the tubing intact and free of kinks.

g. Open the port at the bottom of the urinary collecting bag. This permits all the connections and tubing between the catheter and drainage device to remain closed while permitting you to measure and dispose of accumulated urine.

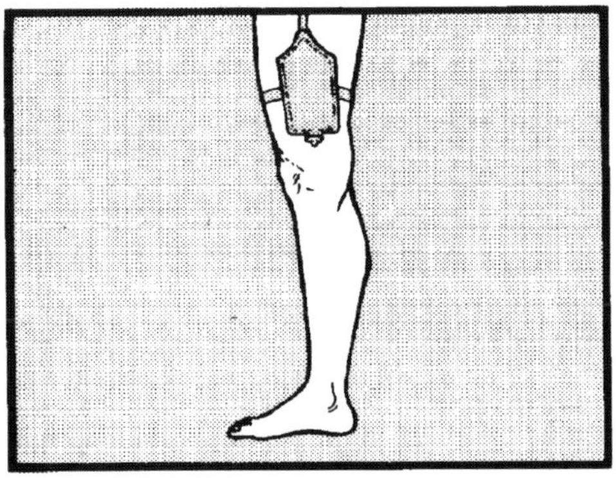

Figure 3-8. Urinary collecting leg bag.

h. Teach the patient to maintain the catheter. Self-care helps the patient develop a feeling of independence and promotes cleanliness. If the patient is ambulatory, instruct him in use of the leg bag. Encourage the patient to intake 2500°cc to 3000 cc of fluid daily.

i. Change the indwelling catheter as necessary or in accordance with local policy.

## 3-9. IRRIGATING AN INDWELLING CATHETER

The purpose of irrigating a catheter is to remove particles that are interfering with the drainage of urine. A catheter that drains well does not need irrigating, except to instill medication. If the patient has a generous fluid intake (2500 cc to 3000 cc of fluid daily), the increase in urine production will dilute the particles that form and irrigate the catheter naturally; thus, invasive procedures may be avoided. Because the drainage system is opened when irrigation takes place, sterile technique is followed.

a. Gather sterile supplies and equipment:

(1) Asepto syringe.

(2) Basin.

(3) Tubing protector.

(4) Gauze moistened with antiseptic.

(5) Sterile normal saline (or other irrigation solution).

b. Using gauze moistened with antiseptic solution, wipe the area where the catheter and tubing join.

**NOTE:** Some catheters have a self-sealing port with a separate lumen through which irrigation solution may be instilled (see figure 3-9). This allows irrigation without separation of the catheter from the collecting device and reduces the possibility of contamination.

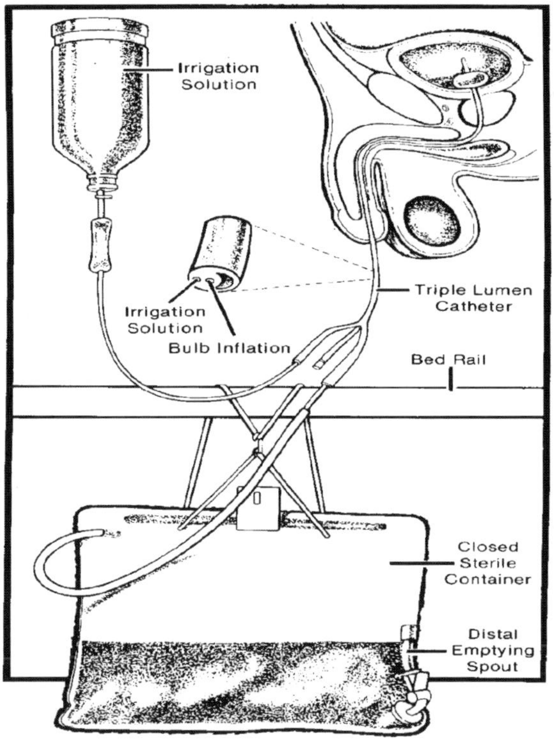


Figure 3-9. Foley triple lumen catheter.

c. Place the sterile tubing protector on the end of the drainage tubing. An alternative is to cover the opening with sterile gauze moistened with antiseptic.

d. Fill the syringe with 30 to 60 cc of solution and insert the syringe tip well into the end of the catheter.

e. Gently compress the ball or end of the syringe to instill the irrigating solution. Do not apply force. Replace the catheter if it cannot be irrigated.

f. Allow the instilled solution to flow back into the basin by gravity.

g. Connect the catheter and drainage tube.

h. Note the total amount of solution used for irrigating and measure the amount of solution returned in the basin. In some cases there is less solution returned than solution instilled. Both amounts must be recorded. The amount that remains will eventually drain into the collection bag.

i. Discard the solution drained into the basin. Replace or protect the irrigating equipment.

j. Record that the irrigation was done, by whom, and the patient's response to the procedure.

## 3-10. REMOVING AN INDWELLING CATHETER

Eventually, a catheter must be removed because the need for it no longer exist or it is crusting and must be changed. The nurse usually removes the catheter.

a. Assemble all supplies and equipment.

(1) 10 cc syringe.

(2) Washcloth and towel.

(3) Exam gloves.

(4) Soap and water.

(5) Chux®

b. Identify the patient and explain the procedure to him. Advise him that there will be a slight burning during removal of the catheter.

c. Provide privacy and assist the female patient into a dorsal recumbent position. The male should be in a supine position. Place Chux® under the patient's buttocks and provide proper draping.

d. Wash your hands and put on exam gloves.

e. Empty the balloon by inserting the barrel of the syringe and withdrawing the amount of fluid used during inflation.

f. Pinch off and gently pull on the catheter near the point where it exits from the meatus.

g. Clean the perineum or penis with soap and water. Dry the area well.

h. Inspect the catheter to be sure no remnants remained in the bladder. If the catheter is not totally intact, report this promptly and save the catheter for further inspection.

i. Empty the drainage bag. Measure the amount of urine and record on the intake and output (I&O) sheet.

j. Remove the gloves and wash your hands.

k. Discard disposable supplies and return reusable supplies and equipment to the appropriate area.

l. Record that the catheter was removed, the time and date and by whom. Note the amount, color, and clarity of the urine in the drainage bag. Also document all patient teaching done and the patient's level of understanding.

m. After removal of the catheter, assess the patient for 24 hours for patterns of urinary elimination. Note the time and amount of the first voided urine. Report any of the following:

(1) Inability to void within 8 to 10 hours.

(2) Frequency, burning, dribbling, or hesitation in starting the stream of urine.

(3) Cloudiness or any other unusual color or characteristic of the urine.

n. Provide a level of fluids similar to the intake when the catheter was in place.

o. Record that the catheter was removed, the date and time, and by whom.

**3-11. CLOSING**

Catheterization can be done without embarrassment and with little discomfort for both the male and female patient. Your observation of urinary output and characteristics of the urine aids in early detection of infection or any other complications. Always remember, you are accountable for responsible care and the safety of the patient.

***Continue with Exercises***

**EXERCISE, LESSON 3**

**NSTRUCTIONS:** To complete this exercise, circle the letter of the response that best answers the question or completes the statement or write the answer in the space provided. After you have completed the all of the exercises, turn to "Solutions to Exercises" at the end of this lesson and check your answers. If you have responded to any of the exercises incorrectly, reread the material referenced after the answer.

1. Catheterization of the urinary bladder is an _______________ procedure for which _______________ equipment is required.

2. Four purposes of urinary catheterization are:

   a. ____________________________________________________________.

   b. ____________________________________________________________.

   c. ____________________________________________________________.

   d. ____________________________________________________________.

3. The French scale (Fr.) is used to denote the size of a catheter. Each unit is roughly equivalent to __________ in diameter.

4. The smaller the number denoting the size of the catheter, the _______________ the catheter.

5. Number 20 Fr. and 22 Fr. catheters are usually used for ______________________.

6. The catheters most commonly used are made of ________________ and have a __________________ to prevent injury to the meatus or urethra.

7. Because catheters are difficult to sterilize, they should be considered __________________ and ________________ after they have been removed.

8. Three types of urinary catheters are:

   a. ______________________________________________.

   b. ______________________________________________.

   c. ______________________________________________.

9. ______________________ is a major risk of catheterization.

10. The catheterization procedure should be done only by trained personnel under __________ conditions.

11. The _________________________ catheter is inserted into the bladder through a small incision above the pubic area.

12. The ___________ catheter is the most commonly used indwelling catheter. It has a balloon at the distal end which is inflated to prevent the catheter from slipping out.

13. When catheterizing a male, you should lubricate the catheter tip at least _______ inches.

14. To cleanse the male meatus, you should use the forceps to hold each cotton ball and swab ____________________________________.

15. To catheterize a male, hold the penis at a _______ angle and gently insert the lubricated catheter into the urinary meatus.

16. When catheterizing a female, you should lubricate the catheter tip at least ______ inches.

17. To catheterize a female, you should use the thumb and forefinger of your ___________________ hand to spread and separate the labia minora. After that hand has touched the patient it is considered to be _________________.

18. To cleanse the female meatus, you should use ________ cotton ball for each stroke, and swab from __________ the meatus downward toward the rectum, then cleanse __________________________________ in the same downward manner.

19. After inserting the catheter into the female meatus, angle it ____________________ as it is advanced.

20. After connecting the catheter to a drainage bag, it should be secured to the female patient's ____________________________.

21. To reduce the possibility of an infection occurring, the patient's perineal area should be cleansed with soap and water _______________________ daily and ______________________________________________________________.

22. To increase urine production and dilute the particles that form in urine, the patient with an indwelling catheter should intake ____________cc to _____________cc of fluid daily.

23. An asepto syringe, basin, tubing protector, sterile solution, and gauze moistened with antiseptic are supplies and equipment used to __________________________ _________________________________________________________.

24. A 10 cc syringe, soap and water, a washcloth and towel, exam gloves, and Chux® are supplies and equipment used to ___________________________________.

25. A ______________________________________________ includes the catheter, a drape, a receptacle to receive urine, materials to cleanse the meatus, a lubricant, a specimen container, and sterile gloves.

Check Your Answers on Next Page

**SOLUTIONS TO EXERCISE, LESSON 3**

1. Aseptic; sterile. (para 3-1)

2. The following in any order.
   To relieve urinary retention.
   To obtain a sterile urine specimen from a female patient.
   To measure the amount of residual urine in the bladder.
   To empty the bladder before, during, or after surgery. (paras 3-2a--d)

3. 33 mm. (para 3-3)

4. Smaller. (para 3-3)

5. Male adult. (para3-3d)

6. Plastic; rounded tip. (para 3-4)

7. Disposable; discarded. (para 3-4)

8. Intermittent.
   Retention or indwelling.
   Supra pubic. (paras 3-4a--c)

9. Infection. (para 3-5)

10. Sterile. (para 3-5)

11. Supra pubic. (para 3-4c)

12. Foley. (para 3-4b(4))

13. Six. (para 3-6f)

14. In a circulate manner from the center of the meatus outward. (para 3-6j)

15. 90°. (para 3-6l)

16. Three. (para 3-7f)

17. Nondominant; contaminated. (para 3-7h)

18. One; above; each side of the meatus. (paras 3-7i--j)

19. Upward. (para 3-7m)

20. Thigh. (para 3-7r and fig. 3-7)

21. Twice; after each bowel movement. (para 3-8b)

22. 2500 cc to 3000 cc. (paras 3-8h, 3-9)

23. Irrigate an indwelling catheter. (paras 3-9a(1)--(5))

24. Remove an indwelling catheter. (paras 3-10a(1)--(5))

25. Disposable indwelling catheter kit. (para 3-5(1))

***End of Lesson 3***

## LESSON ASSIGNMENT

**LESSON 4** Vital Signs

**TEXT ASSIGNMENT** Paragraphs 4-1 through 4-23

**LESSON OBJECTIVES** After completing this lesson, you should be able to:

4-1. Select from a list, three reasons why patients are weighed.

4-2. Select from a list, six principles related to weighing patients.

4-3. Match terms related to body temperature with the correct definition.

4-4. Select from a list, the converted Fahrenheit to Centigrade temperature or vice versa.

4-5. Identify patients who are at risk of hypothermia.

4-6. Identify methods for obtaining an oral, rectal, and axillary temperature.

4-7. Identify precautions, which must be taken when obtaining an oral, rectal, and axillary temperature.

4-8. Identify anatomical sites where a pulse may be taken.

4-9. Select from a list, factors which affect the pulse rate.

4-10. Match terms describing a pulse with the correct definition.

4-11. Match terms related to breathing patterns with the correct definition.

4-12. Match terms related to blood pressure with the correct definition.

4-13. Select from a list, the correct statements relating to a normal adult blood pressure.

4-14. Identify factors, which influence blood pressure values.

4-14. Identify anatomical sites where the blood pressure may be taken.

4-16. Select from a list, principles related to obtaining the blood pressure.

# LESSON 4

# VITAL SIGNS

## 4-1. INTRODUCTION

Soon after a patient arrives on the nursing unit you should begin your nursing assessment. You should take several measurements to establish a baseline for further observations of that patient. Among these measurements are height, weight, and vital signs. The vital signs are the body temperature, the pulse or rate of heartbeats, the respiration or rate of breathing, and the blood pressure. The vital signs are abbreviated TPR and BP for temperature, pulse, respirations and blood pressure. These readings are called vital signs because they all must be present for life to continue.

## 4-2. HEIGHT AND WEIGHT

The patient's height and weight are recorded on admission for several reasons.

a. **Diet Management.** The patient's ideal weight may be determined. The health care team will also be able to monitor weight loss or gain.

b. **Observation of Medical Status.** Taking the patient's height and weight may indicate that the patient is overweight, underweight, or is retaining fluids (edema). The health care team can observe changes in weight caused by specific disease processes and determine the effectiveness of nutrition supplements prescribed to maintain weight.

c. **Calculation of Medication Dosages**. Drug dosage is often prescribed in relation to a patient's weight when a specific blood concentration of the drug is desired. Larger doses may be required in a heavier person.

## 4-3. MEASURING HEIGHT AND WEIGHING THE PATIENT

a. To measure height, have the patient stand on the scale with the back to the measuring bar.

b. Ask the patient to stand straight. Lower the bar so that it lightly touches the top of the patient's head.

c. Record the height in inches or centimeters in accordance with local policy.

d. If the patient cannot stand, obtain an approximate height in bed.

(1) Have the patient lie on his back and stretch as much as possible.

(2) Place a mark on the bottom sheet at the patient's heel and at the top of the patient's head.

(3) Measure between these two marks on the taut bottom sheet.

e. Principles related to weighing the patient.

(1) Weigh the patient before breakfast, at the same time each day.

(2) Use the same scale each time.

(3) Ensure that the scale is properly balanced.

(4) Weigh the patient in the same amount of clothing each day (i.e., hospital gown or pajamas).

(5) Have the patient void before weighing.

(6) Avoid weighing any equipment attached to the patient such as drainage bags or telemetry units. Hold the equipment while actually weighing the patient.

f. A helpless patient may be weighed while lying down on a litter scale. This scale is a sling-type device that looks like a suspended hammock. You will need assistance to place the patient on the scale.

g. Record the patient's weight on the graphic sheet and in the nurses' notes.

## 4-4. TEMPERATURE

Being human, we are homeothermic; we are warm-blooded and maintain body temperature independently of our environment. Our body generates heat as it burns food. It loses heat through the lungs (breathing), through the skin (sweating), and in body discharges (urine, feces, vomitus, or blood). Body temperature is defined as the measure of the heat inside the body: the balance between heat produced and heat lost.

## 4-5. TEMPERATURE REGULATION

a. Heat is produced through the metabolism of food (chemically). Food is used as energy by muscles and glands to generate most of the heat in the body. Heat is also gained (physically) from the environment.

b. During exercise, the muscles become active and the person feels warm. Increasing muscular tone (shivering or gooseflesh) produces heat. The process of digestion also increases body temperature.

c. When a person becomes angry or excited, the adrenal glands become very active and the body warms as a result of the action of certain body chemicals such as epinephrine.

d. Cold, shock, and certain drugs, which depress the nervous system, decreases heat production.

e. The hypothalamus is the body's thermostat. It is located in the central nervous system at the base of the brain. This heat-regulating center in the brain senses any changes in the temperature of blood it receives and makes the appropriate adjustments.

f. Heat loss occurs through the following:

(1) Conduction--direct physical contact with an object.

(2) Convection--when body heat warms surrounding air which rises and is replaced by cooler air.

(3) Radiation--body heat warms surrounding objects without physical contact.

(4) Evaporation--perspiration that is removed from the body surface by change from a liquid to a vapor.

## 4-6. NORMAL BODY TEMPERATURE

A thermometer is placed in the patient's mouth to obtain an oral temperature, in the anal canal to obtain a rectal temperature, and in an axilla (armpit) to obtain an axillary temperature. Table 4-1 shows the average normal temperature for well adults at these various body sites.

| ORAL | RECTAL | AXILLARY |
|---|---|---|
| 98.6° F | 99.5° F | 97.7° F |
| 37.0° C | 37.5° C | 36.5° C |

Table 4-1. Average, normal temperatures for well adults..

a. Temperature is measured on the Fahrenheit (F) or the Celsius (C) scale. The average, normal, oral temperature for an adult is 98.6 degrees Fahrenheit or 37.0 degrees Celsius (old term: centigrade).

b. You can convert Fahrenheit to Celsius or vice versa. To convert Fahrenheit to Celsius, subtract 32 and multiply by 5/9. To convert Celsius to Fahrenheit, multiply by 9/5 and add 32. See Table 4-2 for a conversion chart.

| CELSIUS | FAHRENHEIT |
|---|---|
| 34.0°C | 93.2°F |
| 35.0°C | 95.0°F |
| 36.0°C | 96.8°F |
| 36.5°C | 97.7°F |
| 37.0°C | 98.6°F |
| 37.5°C | 99.5°F |
| 38.0°C | 100.4°F |
| 38.5°C | 101.3°F |
| 39.0°C | 102.2°F |
| 40.0°C | 104.0°F |
| 41.0°C | 105.5°F |
| 42.0°C | 107.6°F |
| 43.0°C | 109.4°F |
| 44.0°C | 111.2°F |

Table 4-2. Celsius/Fahrenheit equivalent temperature.

c. Body temperature may wary by 0.5°F either way and still be within normal limits.

## 4-7. FACTORS WHICH INFLUENCE NORMAL BODY TEMPERATURE

a. Individual metabolism differs. An increase in the emotional state of the patient may increase the temperature.

b. Body temperature is usually lowest in the morning and highest in the late afternoon or evening.

c. Normal temperature for infants and children is usually higher than the normal adult temperature. At birth, heat-regulating mechanisms are not fully developed, so a marked fluctuation in body temperature may occur during the infant's first year of life.

d. In some women, ovulation may be signaled by a slight drop in body temperature 12 to 24 hours before a postovulation rise in temperature of about 0.4°F to 0.8°F.

## 4-8. TERMINOLOGY RELATED TO BODY TEMPERATURE

Body temperature rises when heat production increases or when heat loss decreases; both may be going on at the same time.

a. Everyone has a temperature; when the temperature is elevated, then ***pyrexia*** or a fever is present. A fever is a symptom of some disorder. It often accompanies illness; usually when the body is fighting an infection. An ***antipyretic*** is a fever-reducing agent such as aspirin.

b. A temperature significantly below normal is called ***hypothermia***. Such temperatures often precede normal death. Hypothermia may occur as a result of overexposure to winter elements or to cold water. Accidental hypothermia is life threatening and must be treated immediately. Clinical hypothermia is often used to perform surgical procedures because the lowered body temperature slows metabolism and thus decreases the need for oxygen.

c. The patients most at risk of hypothermia are:

(1) Postoperative patients.

(2) Newborn infants exposed to room temperatures before their body temperature has stabilized.

(3) Elderly or debilitated patients.

## 4-9. TAKING THE TEMPERATURE

Regardless of the type of thermometer or measuring probe used, certain rules apply.

a. The bulb or electronic probe is placed so it will be completely surrounded by body tissues.

b. Multi-use thermometers and temperature probes are covered when used. The cover is removed and discarded after the temperature is taken. Prelubricated covers are used for rectal thermometers.

c. The temperature is recorded on the patient's graphic chart to the even two tenths of a degree (unless the electronic thermometer is used). An electronic thermometer is not calibrated with multiple numbers. It displays only the measured temperature. Record the measured temperature.

## 4-10. TYPES OF THERMOMETERS

a. **Clinical.** The clinical thermometer is a glass bulb containing mercury, with a stem in which the mercury can rise. The stem has lines representing the measuring scale. It must read below normal range before the temperature is taken. It should be rinsed in cold water to avoid distribution of the mercury and breakage. If the thermometer is kept in a chemical solution, dry it with a wipe in a twisting motion starting at the bulb. The clinical thermometer may be oral or rectal.

(1) The oral thermometer has a long, slender bulb. It may also be used for axillary measurement.

(2) The rectal thermometer has a blunt, short, fat bulb. It should not be stored with the oral thermometers.

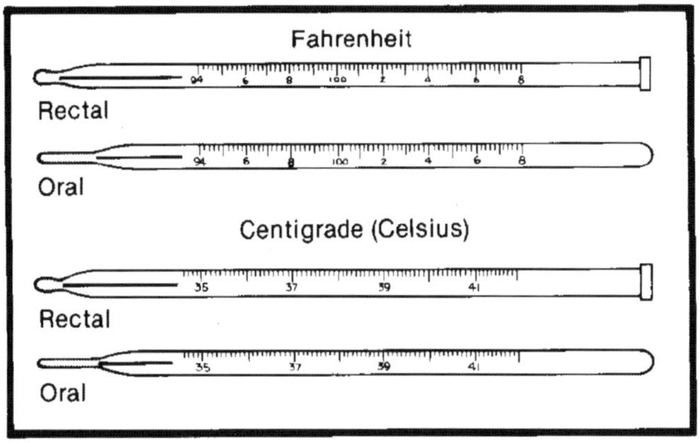


Figure 4-1. Clinical thermometers.

b. **Electronic.** The electronic thermometer is portable and battery operated. It registers the temperature in 10 seconds or less and displays it digitally. It must be fully charged to give an accurate reading, so be sure the thermometer's base is plugged into an electrical outlet between uses. Separate oral and rectal probes are supplied with each unit.

c. **Disposable.** The disposable is single-use and has a sensor at the end of the shaft, which measures the temperature.

d. **Patch.** The thermometer patch is a strip, which contains liquid crystals that change colors as the temperature changes. It is usually placed on the forehead. The scale is adjusted to convert skin-surface temperature to inner-body temperature. The calibration is not as detailed as that of a glass thermometer.

## 4-11. METHODS OF OBTAINING A TEMPERATURE

a. To obtain an oral temperature, place the thermometer in the sublingual pocket and have the patient close his mouth around it. Instruct him not to bite down. Leave the thermometer in place 3 to 4 minutes. If the patient has been eating, drinking, smoking, brushing his teeth, or chewing gum within the past 15 minutes, wait at least 15 minutes to take the temperature.

b. To obtain a rectal temperature, lubricate the bulb and the area up to 1 inch above it. Use a lubricated probe cover with an electronic thermometer. Turn the patient on his side, fold back the bedding and separate the buttocks so that you can easily see the anal opening. Insert the thermometer approximately 1.5 inches into the anus. Hold the thermometer in place for 3 to 4 minutes.

c. To obtain an axillary temperature, place the thermometer in a dry axilla. Keep the arm close to the body to ensure contact with the bulb or probe for 8 to 10 minutes. Axillary is the method of choice for an infant.

d. Precautions.

(1) Oral temperatures are contraindicated for an unconscious patient, for an infant, or when the patient must breathe through the mouth.

(2) The rectal method of obtaining the temperature is contraindicated if the patient has diarrhea, rectal disease, or has recently had rectal surgery.

## 4-12. PULSE

The pulse is the vibration of each wave of blood going through the arteries as the heart beats. The pulse rate is usually equal to heart rate, but may be lower if there is an obstruction of the artery or if the heart rhythm is weak or irregular. You can feel it by placing your fingers over one of the large arteries that lie close to the skin, especially if the artery runs across a bone and has very little soft tissue around it.

a. There are eight common arterial pulse sites. (See figure 4-2).

(1) Radial.

(2) Temporal.

(3) Carotid.

(4) Apical (listening to the heart directly).

(5) Brachial.

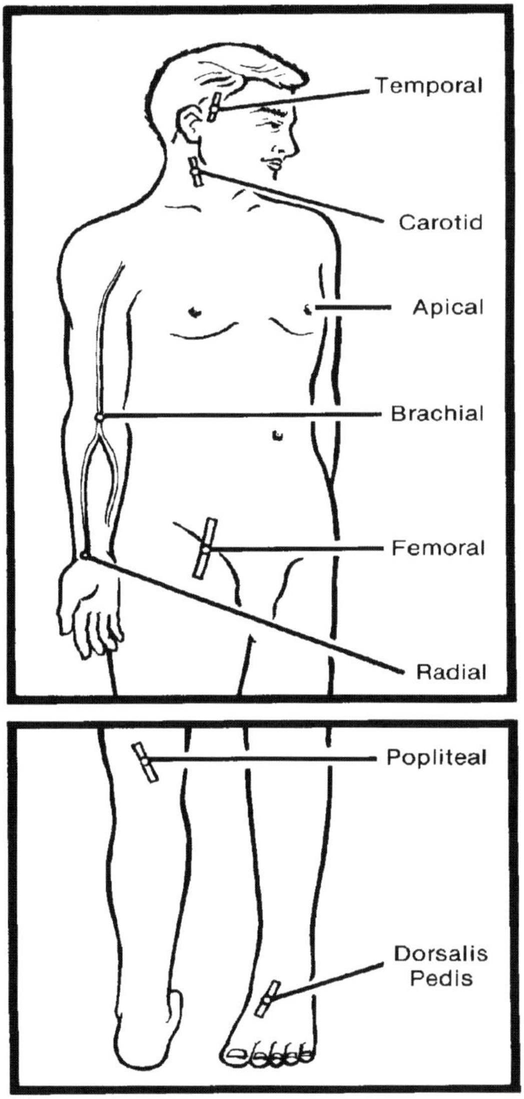


Figure 4 –2. Arterial pulse sites.

(6) Femoral.

(7) Popliteal.

(8) Pedal (dorsalis pedis)

b. The rate that the heart beats varies with the patient's age, size, and weight. The normal rate for an adult is 60 to 80 beats per minute. Women have a slightly higher average rate than men. The pulse of an infant ranges from 120 to 140 beats per minute. Rates for children vary according to the size and the age of the child.

c. Activity affects the pulse rate. Exercise or heavy physical work cause the heart to beat faster and the pulse rate to increase. Excitement, anger, and fear increase the rate. Some drugs, such as caffeine, may also increase the pulse rate. If the patient has a fever, the pulse rate increases in proportion to the body's temperature: the pulse rate goes up about 10 beats for every $1^{\circ}F$ ($0.56^{\circ}C$). These conditions cause a temporary increase in the heartbeat and pulse rate. The heartbeat and pulse rate that is consistently above normal may be a sign of heart disease, heart failure, hemorrhage, an overactive thyroid gland, or some other serious disturbance. The term for an abnormally rapid heartbeat is ***tachycardia***. When the heartbeat is continuously slow, below 60 per minute, the condition is called ***bradycardia***.

## 4-13. DESCRIBING THE PULSE

a. Pulse rate describes ***how often the heart beats***.

b. Pulse volume describes the ***force with which the heart beats***. The volume of the pulse varies with the volume of blood in the arteries, the strength of the heart contractions, and the elasticity of the blood vessels. A ***normal*** pulse can be felt with moderate pressure of the finger. When every beat is easily felt, the pulse is described as ***strong***. When greater pressure exerted by the finger cannot blot out the pulse, it is called ***full or bounding***. A pulse with little force is described as ***weak or thready***.

c. Pulse rhythm is the ***spacing of the heartbeats***. When the intervals between the beats are the same, the pulse is described as ***normal or regular***. When the pulse skips a beat occasionally, it is described as ***intermittent or irregular***. A pulse may be regular in rhythm but irregular in force, with every other beat being weak. To obtain an accurate assessment of the heart rate, the pulse is counted by listening directly to the heart (apical pulse).

## 4-14. FACTORS, WHICH AFFECT THE PULSE RATE

The pulse rate is an indicator of how fast the heart beats. The pulse rate is affected by several factors.

a. **Age.** A normal pulse for infants range from 90 to 170 and the rate gradually decreases up to age 14 when it is equal to the normal adult pulse rate of 60 to 100.

b. **Body Build and Size.** A short, fat person may have a higher rate than a tall, slender person.

c. **Blood Pressure.** As the blood pressure decreases, the pulse will frequently increase.

d. **Medications.** Stimulants will increase the pulse rate; depressants will decrease the pulse rate.

e. **Exercise and Muscular Activity.** An increase in pulse rate will occur with increased activity to meet increased oxygen and nutrient demands. A regular aerobic exercise program can lower the resting pulse. A person, who exercises a great deal, such as an athlete, will develop bradycardia that is a normal, health condition. The body slows the heartbeat to compensate for the greater volume of blood pumped with each beat.

f. **Food Intake.** Digestion increases the pulse slightly.

g. **Elevated Body Temperature.** The pulse increases approximately 10 beats per minute for every 1 F (0.56° C) increase in body temperature. These conditions cause a temporary increase in the heartbeat and pulse.

h. **Emotional Status.** Fear, anger, and anxiety will all increase the pulse rate.

i. **Pain.** When the patient is in pain, the pulse rate will increase.

## 4-15. MEASURING THE PULSE

a. **Measuring a Radial Pulse.**

(1) Wash your hands to prevent the spread of infection.

(2) Supporting the patient's arm and hand with the palm down, press the first, second, and third finger of your dominant hand gently against the radius bone until you feel the contraction and expansion of the artery with each heartbeat. Do not use your thumb; it has a strong pulse of its own and you may be counting your pulse.

(3) Count the pulsations for 30 seconds using a watch with a second hand or digital display to time yourself. Multiply the count by 2 to determine the rate for 1 minute. If the pulse is abnormal in any way, count for a full minute to get a more accurate reading.

(4) The pulse rate may also be determined by the electronic vital signs monitor (see figure 4-3).

(5) If there is any doubt about the rhythm or rate of the heart, take an apical pulse.

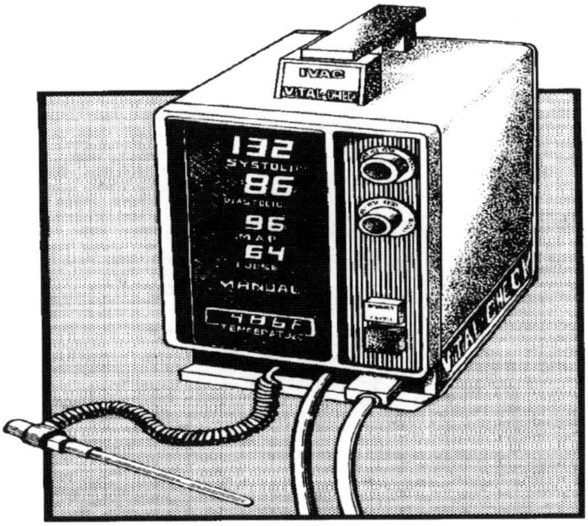


Figure 4-3. Electronic vital signs monitor.

b. **Measuring an Apical Pulse.**

(1) Warm the stethoscope in your hands. A cold stethoscope may surprise the patient and alter the pulse rate.

(2) Place the stethoscope at the apex (pointed end) of the heart, in the left center of the chest, just below the nipple. The pulse can usually be heard best at the apex.

(3) Count the pulse for one full minute.

c. **Measuring the Apical-Radial Pulse.**

(1) If the apical-radial (A-R) pulse is ordered by the physician, two nurses carry out the procedure together.

(2) Using the same watch, one nurse counts the patient's apical pulse for 1 minute while the other nurse counts the radial pulse for 1 minute. One nurse gives the signal to start counting, and both start at the same time. The two figures are identified and charted (A-R pulse 76/72, for example). Normally, these two readings should be the same. If there is a difference, it is called the pulse deficit.

**NOTE:** An apical pulse will never be lower than the radial pulse.

## 4-16. RESPIRATION

Respiration is the process that brings oxygen into the body and removes carbon dioxide waste. The exchange occurs in the lungs. Respiration occurs in two phases: internal and external.

a. Internal respiration is the process by which oxygen is taken from the bloodstream into the cell and carbon dioxide is removed from the cell to the bloodstream.

b. External respiration refers to delivery of oxygen to the lungs so that it can be taken into the bloodstream. External respiration (breathing) has two components: Inspiration, the process of taking air into the lungs; and expiration, expelling air from the lungs.

c. It is the rate of external respiration that is measured. The normal adult rate is 14 to 20 breaths per minute. Women have a more rapid rate than men. Newborns have a normal rate of about 40. Children have a normal rate of 25 to 30.

d. Respiration is controlled and regulated by the respiratory center in the brain and by the amount of carbon dioxide in the blood. Respiration is involuntary and automatic. You can control the action of your breathing to some extent, but only for a limited time. If automatic breathing does not occur, a breathing disorder exists.

## 4-17. BREATHING PATTERNS

a. Normal breathing is relaxed, effortless, and regular.

b. Rapid breathing is a rate above 20 breaths per minute, associated with increased activity or a disease process. The medical term is ***tachypnea***.

c. Slow breathing is a rate below 14. It may also be described as shallow if the patient takes in and breathes out small amounts of air.

d. Difficult breathing describes when a person is making a definite effort to get more oxygen and get rid of carbon dioxide. ***Dyspnea*** is the term for difficult breathing. Dyspnea is also the term used for painful breathing, a subjective pattern, which must be stated by the patient. Dyspnea may be a temporary condition, such as when a runner gasps at the end of a race or when a person pants "to get his breathe" after climbing stairs. In some diseases, such as pneumonia, emphysema, or some types of heart conditions, breathing difficulty is more or less constant. Signs of breathing difficulties are: heaving of the chest and the abdomen, and ***cyanosis*** (a bluish tinge in the skin).

e. ***Orthopnea*** is the term used if the patient can breathe only when in an upright position.

f. ***Apnea*** is the absence of respirations.

g. ***Cheyne-Stokes*** is the term for cycles of breathing characterized by deep, rapid breaths for about 30 seconds, followed by absence of respirations for 10 to 30 seconds. Cheyne-Stokes respirations constitute a serious symptom and usually precedes death in cerebral hemorrhage, uremia, or heart disease.

## 4-18. BLOOD PRESSURE

Two things determine the blood pressure: the rate and force of the heartbeat and the ease with which the blood flows into the small branches of the arteries. When the heart rate or force is increased by exertion or illness, blood pressure increases. If the volume of blood within the circulatory system is reduced (as in hemorrhage), and other factors remain the same, blood pressure decreases.

a. Blood pressure is the pressure exerted by the blood on the walls of the blood vessels within the systemic arterial system. Normal systolic pressure for a young adult is 100 to 120 mmHg (millimeters of mercury); diastolic pressure is about 80. Blood pressure increases gradually with age. Normal systolic pressure for a person 60 years of age is 130 to 140. ***Hypertension*** is blood pressure above normal limits (above 140/90); it is a sign of a circulatory problem. ***Hypotension*** is blood pressure below normal limits (below 90/60) and may indicate shock. See table 4-3.

| | |
|---|---|
| **SYSTOLIC** | **100 to 140 mmHg** |
| **DIASTOLIC** | **60 to 90 mmHG** |

Table 4-3. Normal range of adult blood pressure.

b. ***Systolic*** blood pressure is greatest. It is the pressure against the wall of the blood vessels following ventricular contraction. Using the auscultatory (listening) method, the systolic blood pressure is recorded at the highest point at which two consecutive beats are heard (Korotkoff sounds).

c. ***Diastolic*** blood pressure is lowest. It is the pressure against the blood vessels when the heart is relaxed before it begins to contract again.

d. The ***mean arterial pressure (MAP)*** denotes the average pressure within the arteries. An electronic vital signs monitor can determine and display an accurate average pressure or MAP.

e. Shock or other difficulty is usually indicated by a systolic reading of 80 or less. A diastolic reading over 100 is usually considered dangerously high.

## 4-19. MEASURING BLOOD PRESSURE

Blood pressure is usually measured indirectly using a ***stethoscope*** and an instrument called the ***sphygmomanometer***. The most common site is the arm just above the antecubital area, using the brachial artery. Blood pressure may be measured directly by means of a catheter or probe inserted into a blood vessel or the heart.

a. **Direct Measurement.**

(1) One means of direct blood pressure measurement is to place a special tube in a vein and monitor central venous pressure (CVP). Central venous pressure may be used to determine fluid needs in shock, hemorrhage, or severe burns, to detect pulmonary edema, and to determine the extent of circulatory overload.

(2) Another method of direct blood pressure measurement is internal or invasive monitoring. A large, flexible catheter, such as a Swan-Ganz catheter measures pressures within the heart itself.

b. **Indirect Measurement.** The sphygmomanometer (often called a blood pressure apparatus) includes a wide, cloth-covered rubber cuff with two rubber tubes extending from it. One tube is connected to a bulb air pump that has a valve, which can be opened or closed. The other tube is connected to a glass cylinder containing mercury (mercury manometer) or to a dial (aneroid manometer), which attaches to the arm wrap. You obtain the indirect blood pressure reading with the manometer by listening to the heartbeat with a stethoscope.

(1) Cleanse the stethoscope and earpiece with an alcohol wipe before and after the procedure (unless you use your own stethoscope).

(2) Have the patient lie down or rest comfortably in a chair with the arm supported and the palm turned upward to expose the brachial artery on the inside of the elbow.

(3) Let the air out of the cuff. Wrap the cuff firmly around the arm, just far enough above the elbow to leave the space over the brachial artery free, and fasten the clip or Velcro closure.

(4) Find the pulse in the artery and place the stethoscope over the spot where you can feel the strongest pulsations.

(5) Pump the manometer bulb to 20 mm above a possible systolic pressure. Release the valve on the manometer bulb to gradually release air from the cuff.

(6) Note the level on the mercury column or dial at which you first hear a heartbeat. This is the systolic pressure.

(7) Continue gradually releasing air from the cuff. Note the point on the mercury column or dial at which the heartbeat cannot be heard, or at which there is a distinct change in the sound. This is the diastolic pressure.

(8) Release the remaining air from the cuff. Record the blood pressure reading on the patient's chart by writing the systolic pressure above the diastolic pressure. Use only even numbers.

EXAMPLE: BP $\frac{120}{80}$ or 120/80

c. **Alternate Site for Measurement.** If it is impossible to measure the blood pressure in the arm, the leg is used. When blood pressure is taken in the leg, the popliteal space (popliteal artery) is used, and the cuff is applied above the knee. If you measure the blood pressure at any site other than the arm, use the appropriate size cuff and indicate the site on the chart.

d. **Electronic Blood Pressure Apparatus.** The cuff of the electronic blood pressure apparatus is applied and manipulated in basically the same manner as with the mercury or aneroid manometer. The cuff is usually inflated and deflated automatically. It is important to place the microphone under the cuff so the arrow that indicates "artery" is in the correct location. Systolic and diastolic pressures will be printed out on the screen within a few seconds.

## 4-20. FACTORS WHICH INFLUENCE BLOOD PRESSURE VALUES

a. **Age.** Children normally have lower blood pressure at birth (80/60), which gradually increases until the age of 18 when it becomes equal to the normal adult pressure. Older adults frequently have higher blood pressure due to a decrease in blood vessel elasticity.

b. **Sex.** Men have higher blood pressure than women of the same age.

c. **Body Build.** Blood pressure is usually elevated in an obese person.

d. **Exercise.** Muscular exertion will temporarily elevate the blood pressure. A regular exercise program can eventually decrease the resting blood pressure.

e. **Pain.** Physical discomfort will usually elevate the blood pressure.

f. **Emotional Status.** Fear, worry, or excitement can elevate the blood pressure.

g. **Disease States and Medication.** Some disease conditions and/or the medications influence the blood pressure.

## 4-21. PRINCIPLES RELATED TO OBTAINING THE BLOOD PRESSURE

a. The patient's arm must be at the level of the heart. If the arm is below the heart, false elevated pressures are obtained. If the arm is above the heart, false lowered blood pressures are obtained.

b. The arm should be supported during the entire procedure to prevent elevation due to muscle contractions used to maintain the position.

c. The cuff and stethoscope should be placed directly on the skin. Light pressure should be applied when placing the stethoscope over the artery.

d. The cuff should be quickly deflated to zero, once the last measurement is heard. Wait a minimum of 30 seconds before measuring the blood pressure again.

## 4-22. THE GRAPHIC SHEET

a. A graphic sheet is maintained so that all vital sign readings are easily accessible to members of the health care team. Each reading is recorded as a dot in the proper space, with lines connecting the dots. Readings throughout the patient's illness are indicated across the page in unbroken lines. The form used to graphically record the patient's vital signs in a United States (US) Army hospital is SF 511, Clinical Record--Vital Signs Record.

b. Recording data.

(1) Enter the patient's identification data in the space at the bottom of the form.

(2) Number the "Hospital Day" line of blocks with the day of admission as one, and continue consecutively. Use the "Post-op Day" line as applicable. The day of surgery is the operative day. The day following surgery is noted as the first post-operative day.

(3) Label the day/hour blocks properly.

(4) Represent temperature by dots placed between the columns and rows, and joined by straight lines. If the temperature is other than oral, indicate so by (R) for rectal or (A) for axillary.

(5) Show pulse by use of a circle connected by straight lines.

(6) Enter the respiration and blood pressure on the indicated rows below the graphic portion.

(7) Record frequent blood pressure readings on the form's graphic portion by entering an "X" between the columns and rows of dots, at points equivalent to systolic and

diastolic levels. Connect the two with a vertical solid line.

(8) Use blank lines at the bottom of the sheet to record special data such as the 24-hour total of the patient's intake and output.

**4-23. CLOSING**

Measuring and recording vital signs is not complicated; however, these are important tasks because these measurements are indicators of functions, which are necessary to sustain life. The patient's current vital signs can be compared with those previously obtained or with normal values and changes in health can be detected and treated quickly.

***Continue with Exercises***

**EXERCISE, LESSON 4**

**INSTRUCTIONS:** To complete this exercise, circle the letter of the response that best answers the question or completes the statement or write the answer in the space provided. After you have completed the all of the exercises, turn to "Solutions to Exercises" at the end of this lesson and check your answers. If you have responded to any of the exercises incorrectly, reread the material referenced after the answer.

1. Vital signs are:

   a. ______________________________.

   b. ______________________________.

   c. ______________________________.

   d. ______________________________.

2. One of the measurements taken to establish a baseline for further observation of the patient is his weight. Three reasons for weighing the patient are:

   a. ______________________________.

   b. ______________________________.

   c. ______________________________.

3. Six principles related to weighing the patient are

   a. ______________________________.

   b. ______________________________.

   c. ______________________________.

   d. ______________________________.

   e. ______________________________.

   f. ______________________________.

4. A helpless patient may be weighed while lying down on a ________________.

5. Bold temperature is defined as the measure of heat inside the body or the balance between ______________________________________________

6. Body heat is lost through:

   a. ________________, which is direct physical contact with an object.

   b. __________________ when body heat warms the surrounding air.

   c. __________________ when body heat warms surrounding objects without physical contact.

   d. __________________ when perspiration changes from a liquid to a vapor.

7. The average, normal, oral temperature for an adult is _______ °F or _______ °C.

8. To convert Celcius to Fahrenheit, you should __________________ and __________.

9. If the patient has a temperature of 37.5° C, the converted Fahrenheit temperature would be:

   a. 97.7°.

   b. 99.5°.

   c. 97.5°.

10. Four factors, which influence normal body temperature, are:

   a. ______________________________________________.

   b. ______________________________________________.

   c. ______________________________________________.

   d. ______________________________________________.

11. When the patient has an elevated temperature, _____________ (a fever) is present.

12. The medical term for a temperature below normal is _____________________.

13. Patients most at risk for hypothermia are:

    a. __________________________________________________.

    b. __________________________________________________.

    c. __________________________________________________.

14. To obtain an oral temperature, place the thermometer in the __________________ for _______________________ minutes.

15. To obtain a rectal temperature, insert the thermometer into the anal opening __________ inches for ________________ minutes.

16. To obtain an axillary temperature, place the thermometer in a ___________ axilla for ____________________ minutes.

17. Certain precautions must be taken when obtaining a temperature. The rectal method is contraindicated if the patient has:

    a. __________________________________________________.

    b. __________________________________________________.

    c. __________________________________________________.

18. There are eight common arterial pulse sites; list three of these sites.

    a. ________________________________________________.

    b. ________________________________________________.

    c. ________________________________________________.

19. The pulse rate indicates how often the heart beats. ____________________ means that the heartbeat is abnormally rapid. When the heartbeat is continuously slow, the condition is called ________________________________.

20. A normal pulse can be felt with moderate pressure of the finger. When greater pressure exerted by the finger cannot blot out the pulse, it is called ____________________________. A pulse with little force is described as ________________________________.

21. Body build and size are factors, which affect the pulse rate. A short, fat person will probably have a ____________________ pulse rate than a tall, slender person.

22. The normal breathing pattern is relaxed, effortless, and regular. When breathing is rapid, the term used is ________________________________.

23. ________________ is the medical term used when breathing is difficult or painful.

24. ____________________________ is the term for cycles of deep, rapid breaths for about 30 seconds, followed by absence of respiration for 10 to 30 seconds. This pattern of respiration sometimes precedes death.

25. Normal blood pressure for a young adult is about 120/80. ____________________ is blood pressure above 140/90. If the blood pressure is below 90/60, the patient has ______________________________ and may be in shock.

26. List five factors, which influence blood pressure values:

a. ____________________________________________.

b. ____________________________________________.

c. ____________________________________________.

d. ____________________________________________.

e. ____________________________________________.

27. The most common site for measuring blood pressure is the _______________, just above the antecubital area, using the___________________________ artery.

28. List two principles related to obtaining the blood pressure.

a. _________________________________________________________________.

b. _________________________________________________________________.

*Check Your Answers on Next Page*

## SOLUTIONS TO EXERCISE, LESSON 4

1. Temperature.
   Pulse.
   Respiration.
   Blood pressure. (para 4-1)

2. Diet management.
   Observation of medical status.
   Calculation of medication dosages. (paras 4-2a--c)

3. Weigh him before breakfast.
   Use the same scales.
   Assure that the scales are properly balanced.
   Weigh him in the same amount of clothing.
   Have him void before you weigh him.
   Avoid weighing any equipment attached to him. (paras 4-3e(1)--(6))

4. Litter scales. (para 4-3f)

5. Heat produced and heat lost. (para 4-4)

6. a. Conduction.
   b. Convection.
   c. Radiation.
   d. Evaporation. (paras 4-5f(1)--(4))

7. 98.6°F; 37.0°C. (para 4-6a, Table 4-1)

8. Multiply by 9/5; add 32. (para 4-6b)

9. b (para 4-6b, Table 4-2)

10. Individual metabolism differs.
    Body temperature is lower in the morning and higher in the evening.
    Normal temperature for infants and children is higher than normal adult temperature.
    Ovulation in some women cause a slight rise followed by a drop in body temperature. (paras 4-7a--d)

11. Pyrexia. (para 4-8a)

12. Hypothermia. (para 4-8b)

13. Postoperative patients.
    Newborn infants.
    Elderly or debilitated patients. (paras 4-8c(1)--(3))

14. Sublingual pocket; 3 to 4. (para 4-11a)

15. 1.5; 3 to 4. (para 4-11b)

16. Dry; 8 to 10. (para 4-11c)

17. Diarrhea.
    Rectal disease.
    Recently had rectal surgery. (para 4-11d)

18. Any **three** of the following is correct:
    Temporal.
    Carotid.
    Apical.
    Brachial.
    Femoral.
    Radial.
    Popliteal.
    Dorsalis pedis. (para 4-12)

19. Tachycardia; bradycardia. (para 4-12c)

20. Full or bounding; weak or thready. (para 4-13b)

21. Higher. (para 4-14b)

22. Tachypnea. (para 4-17b)

23. Dyspnea. (para 4-17d)

24. Cheyne-Stokes. (para 4-17g)

25. Hypertension; hypotension. (para 4-18a)

26. Any **five** of the following is correct:
    Age.
    Sex.
    Body build.
    Exercise.
    Pain.
    Emotional status.
    Disease state and medication. (paras 4-20a--g)

27. Arm; brachial. (para 4-19)

28. Any **two** of the following is correct:
The patient's arm must be at the level of the heart.
The arm should be supported during the entire procedure.
The cuff and stethoscope should be placed directly on the skin.
The cuff should be quickly deflated to zero, once the last measurement is heard.
(paras 4-21a--d)

***End of Lesson 4***

## LESSON ASSIGNMENT

**LESSON 5** Diet Therapy

**TEXT ASSIGNMENT** Paragraphs 5-1 through 5-13

**LESSON OBJECTIVES** After completing this lesson, you should be able to:

5-1. Select from a list six factors which influence eating patterns.

5-2. Identify factors, which may alter a hospitalized patient's eating patterns.

5-3. Identify factors, which may alter a patient's food intake due to illness.

5-4. Identify reasons that hospitalized patients are at risk of being malnourished.

5-5. Identify nursing interventions, which may help, the patient meets his or her nutritional needs.

5-6 Identify the responsibilities of the practical nurse in relation to diet therapy.

5-7. Identify six reasons for therapeutic diets.

5-8. Select a specialized diet when given a description of the diet contents.

5-9. Identify nursing interventions, which may prepare the patient for meals.

**SUGGESTION** After studying the assignment, complete the exercises at the end of this lesson. These exercises will help you to achieve the lesson objectives.

# LESSON 5

# DIET THERAPY

## 5-1. INTRODUCTION

Food is essential to life. To sustain life, the nutrients in food must perform three functions within the body: build tissue, regulate metabolic processes, and provide a source of energy. A proper diet is essential to good health. A well-nourished person is more likely to be well developed, mentally and physically alert, and better able to resist infectious diseases than one who is not well nourished. Proper diet creates a healthier person and extends the years of normal bodily functions. Diet therapy is the application of nutritional science to promote human health and treat disease.

## 5-2. FACTORS WHICH INFLUENCE EATING PATTERNS

We all eat certain foods for reasons other than good nutrition and health. Our eating patterns develop as part of our cultural and social traditions and are influenced by our life style and life situation. It is important for the nurse to understand factors, which influence food choice and eating patterns.

a. **Social Aspects.** Most people prefer to eat with someone, and the patient is probably used to eating meals with his family. In the hospital he is served his food on a tray and left alone. Poor nutrition may be the result.

b. **Emotional Aspects.** The patient may feel guilty for not eating all the food served, or may overeat just because the food is there. The patient may overeat because he or she feels sad, lonely, or depressed or may refuse to eat for the same reasons. Certain foods may be considered "for babies." Some foods may be used as rewards."

c. **Food Fads and Fallacies.** These are scientifically unsubstantiated, misleading notions or beliefs about certain foods that may persist for a time in a given community or society. Many people follow fad diets or the practice of eating only certain foods. Food fads fall into four basic groups: Food cures, harmful foods, food combinations that restore health or reduce weight, and natural foods that meet body needs and prevent disease.

d. **Financial Considerations.** The patient's financial status has a great bearing on eating patterns. Most people in the United States can afford a diet, which includes a variety of foods and a sufficient number of calories. However, many Americans consume an excessive amount of fat and sodium. Excess fat consumption has been shown to be related to the development of heart disease. Excess sodium consumption may be a problem for some patients with hypertension. Many Americans with lower incomes consume a great percentage of their calories in the form of fat, since fat is the least expensive nutrient (when compared to carbohydrate and protein) and provides for greater satiety (feeling of "fullness" after eating) than both carbohydrate and protein."

e. **Physical Condition.** The patient may not feel well enough or strong enough to eat. Encourage the patient to eat without forcing him to do so. Encourage him to feed himself, so that he will not feel helpless.

f. **Cultural Heritage.** Food preferences are closely tied to culture and religion. Understanding these preferences will enable you to assist the patient in reaching and maintaining good nutritional health.

(1) African-Americans. Food habits may be based on West Indian, African, or regional American influences. The majority of African-Americans are lactose intolerant and avoid milk but can tolerate cheese, yogurt, and ice cream. African-Americans who have been in the US for many generations have similar eating patterns to other Americans. Their diets are rich in fat, salt, sugar, and starches. Those who have recently immigrated to the US eat the staple rice and bean combination, yams, and tropical fruits.

(2) Hispanic-Americans. The Hispanic population is thought to be 60 percent Mexican, 18 percent Central and South American, 15 percent Puerto Rican, and 7 percent Cuban. They are a varied group having different food habits.

(a) Mexican-Americans eat tortillas, rice and beans with most meals. Meats are heavily spiced, and often chopped or ground. Adults use limited amounts of milk and milk products, but enjoy sweet baked desserts, sweetened beverages such as hot chocolate and carbonated drinks.

(b) Puerto Ricans tend to adopt American food habits. Traditional meals include white rice cooked with lard and served with beans. Some practice the "hot-cold" theory in the treatment of illness with food.

(c) Cuban-Americans use rice and beans extensively and meat is served if income is sufficient. Children drink milk but adults use milk only in coffee.

(3) Chinese-Americans. A common dietary principle is "Fan-tsai." Fan is the grain and tsai are the vegetables or other items served at the meal. Chinese-Americans obtain 80 percent of their calories from grains and 20 percent from vegetables, fruits, animal protein, and fats. Most adults dislike milk and cheese. Lactose intolerance is common.

(4) Japanese-American. Most Japanese-American's eating habits are Westernized. Traditional meals are light and little animal fat is used. The major starch used is rice. Meals contain fish, soup, fresh or pickled vegetables, and tea.

(5) Indian-Americans. Eating patterns vary, depending upon the religion, and the province and climate from which the Indian-American came. If from northern India, wheat is the primary grain used and meat dishes are popular. If from southern India, rice is the primary grain used, the food is highly spiced, and the person will usually be a vegetarian because of Hindu beliefs. Sweets are very sweet and eaten often. Most Indian-American's eat only two meals daily. Only the right hand is used for eating. Women eat only after men and children have eaten, even if they are ill. Traditional fads and fallacies result in a high rate of stillbirths, low birth weight infants, and a high maternal death rates.

(6) Native-Americans. Because about 200 different tribes of Native Americans exist in the United States, each with its own language, folkways, religion, mores, and patterns of interpersonal relationships, caution needs to be taken in generalizing about Native American culture and food preferences. Various tribal groups differ in their traditional values and beliefs. Each tribe assigns symbolic meanings to foods or other substances. At least one-third of the Native American population is poverty-stricken. Associated with this income level are poor living conditions and malnutrition.

## 5-3. RELIGION

Cultural and religious practices are often intertwined. Many people refrain from eating certain foods, or eat specific foods in certain combinations, because of their religious beliefs. There are some major religious customs related to diet that, as a nurse, you must be aware of.

a. **Hindu.** Most Hindus are lacto-ovo vegetarians. They do not use stimulants such as alcohol or coffee.

b. **Moslem (Islam).** Meat and poultry must be slaughtered according to strict rules. Moslems do not eat pork or pork products. They do not drink alcoholic beverages. They do drink tea. Moslems fast for one month each year, avoiding food from dawn until after dark.

c. **Jewish (Orthodox).** Orthodox Jews do not eat pork, shellfish, or scavenger fish. They do eat beef, veal, lamb, mutton, goat, venison, chicken, turkey, goose, and pheasant. Meat must be slaughtered by a ritual method. Meat and milk may not be served at the same meal. Meat and dairy foods must be prepared in separate containers and with separate utensils. Certain days of fasting are observed, but a rabbi may excuse an elderly or ill patient.

d. **Mormon.** Mormons do not drink alcohol, coffee, tea, or caffeine containing carbonated beverages. They do not use extremely hot or cold foods (no ice in beverages).

e. **Roman Catholic.** Catholics may voluntarily abstain from eating meat on Fridays and during Lent. They do not eat or drink (except water) before taking Holy Communion. They fast on Good Friday and Ash Wednesday, but a priest may excuse the elderly or an ill patient.

f. **Seventh Day Adventists.** Seventh Day Adventists do not drink alcohol, coffee, or tea. They are usually lacto-ovo vegetarians.

## 5-4. THE VEGETARIAN

a. Because of the dangers of too much animal protein resulting in health problems or for ecological reasons, many people have chosen to be vegetarians. They do not eat any type of meat. Some vegetarian diets are stricter than others.

(1) Lacto vegetarians eat plant foods and dairy products. They do not eat eggs.

(2) Ovo vegetarians eat plant foods and eggs. They do not eat dairy products.

(3) Lacto-ovo vegetarians eat plant foods, dairy products, and eggs.

(4) Fruitarians consume a diet that consists chiefly of fruits, nuts, olive oil, and honey. They do not eat any animal products.

(5) Vegans eat only plant foods.

b. The greatest concern in the vegetarian diet is attaining adequate amounts of complete protein. This is easy in the lacto-ovo vegetarian diet, but difficult for the vegan. The most efficient protein available is that found in dairy products, eggs, and fish. Among the sources of protein that can be used most efficiently by the body, meat actually ranks third. The second best supply of efficient protein is legumes, soybeans, nuts, and brown rice.

c. Complete proteins are needed to sustain life and to promote growth. Incomplete protein sources can be combined to become a complete protein.

(1) Grain may be combined with brewer's yeast, with milk and cheese, with nuts and milk or legumes. Examples are cereal and milk, a peanut butter sandwich and milk or yogurt, a cheese sandwich; rice cooked in milk, and baked beans with nut bread.

(2) Grain with dried beans or wheat germ and nuts, grain with egg, and grain with cheese. Examples are a poached egg on toast, macaroni and cheese, and a tortilla with cheese.

(3) Beans, legumes (peas, lentils), rice or soybeans (tofu) with milk, nuts, or eggs.

d. Vegans should eat at least two of the following at the same meal in order to provide all essential amino acids:

(1) Grains or nuts and seeds.

(2) Dried beans or tofu.

(3) Wheat germ.

e. Whole-wheat grains and cereals are preferred in vegetarian diets. Other foods must be added to the protein sources to supply vitamins and minerals. Vegetarian diets are often deficient in calcium, iron, zinc, vitamin D, iodine, and riboflavin. Vitamin B12 is probably missing entirely. Supplements of these substances often need to be taken.

## 5-5. FACTORS WHICH ALTER A HOSPITALIZED PATIENT'S EATING PATTERNS

The meals served in a hospital cannot accommodate all social and cultural variations in food habits. However, meals can be individualized to assure that patients are provided with foods that are acceptable to them, but still within the restrictions of their diet. A meal, no matter how carefully planned, serves its purpose only if it is eaten. Many factors alter a patient's eating patterns during hospitalization.

a. The forced menu of available foods.

b. Isolation from family and significant others.

c. Restriction in activity.

d. A forced eating schedule.

## 5-6. FACTORS IN ILLNESS WHICH MAY ALTER FOOD INTAKE

Nutrition plays an important part in a patient's overall condition. A person who is ill may need help in meeting his basic needs for adequate nutrition. Certain factors in illness may alter food intake.

a. The disease processes. The patient's ability to ingest food is dependent upon the condition of his mouth and oral structures, and his ability to swallow. Impairment of any of these components will interfere with eating.

b. Drug therapy, which may alter the patient's appetite.

c. Anxiety about his illness.

d. Loneliness.

e. Diet restrictions. In many disease conditions, a special diet is an important part of therapy. In addition to educating the patient about the diet, you should help him to adapt to the diet and enjoy the food that he can have.

f. Changes in usual activity level. Exercise has been reported to increase, decrease, or have no effect on food intake. Although food intake is decreased immediately after exercise, habitual moderate exercise over a long period of time promotes increased food intake.

## 5-7. REASONS FOR HOSPITALIZED PATIENTS BEING AT RISK OF MALNUTRITION

a. The effect of the disease on metabolism. Most illnesses and diseases increase the need for nutrients. For example, one of the first symptoms of an infectious disease is loss of appetite and decreased tolerances for food. But, the infection and possible fever increase the metabolic rate and the actual nutrient requirements.

b. The disease may cause problems with absorption. An abnormality in either secretion or motility affects not only digestion but also optimal absorption. Motility is the movement of food through the digestive tract.

(1) Alterations in motility in the esophagus or stomach may result in symptoms of indigestion and vomiting. Increased motility of the gastric contents through the small and large intestines results in decreased absorption and diarrhea.

(2) Conditions that increase motility of the small intestine primarily affect absorption.

c. The anxiety and stress of being ill may reduce the patient's appetite.

d. The treatment may cause problems with intake, digestion, or absorption. The decreased desire to eat may be caused by impaired ability to taste food because of medication, bloating resulting from decreased peristalsis in the gastrointestinal tract following surgery, or nausea resulting from chemotherapy. Withholding food for various tests and procedures, or restricting the patient's intake may affect his appetite.

## 5.8. NURSING INTERVENTIONS WHICH HELP THE PATIENT MEET NUTRITIONAL NEEDS

Mealtime is an important event in the patient's long day and the patient's diet is an integral part of the total treatment plan. Certain nursing interventions may help the patient meet his or her nutritional needs.

a. Consider the patient's food preferences as much as possible. Encourage the patient to fill out the selective menu, so that preferred foods will be served.

b. Provide the patient with assistance in selecting the appropriate foods from the menu. The use of selective menus has improved food acceptance in most hospitals.

c. Order and deliver the patient's tray promptly when it has been delayed while he was undergoing tests or procedures.

d. Feed or assist the patient as necessary. Even patients, who can feed themselves, may need assistance in opening milk cartons, cutting meat, and spreading butter on bread.

e. Discuss the advantages of following the diet. Explain to the patient why he will feel better and heal faster. For some diseases or disorders, the patient may be required to follow a special diet during the period of illness or the remainder of his life.

(1) A high protein diet is essential to repair tissues in any condition, which involves healing, such as recovery from surgery or burns.

(2) A person with diabetes must adhere to a diet controlled in calories, carbohydrates, protein, and fat.

(3) A person with hypertension may require a diet restricted in sodium.

f. Inform the dietitian or food service specialist of any special needs the patient may have. A patient who has lost his teeth and has difficulty chewing will need modifications in the consistency of the food he eats.

g. Visit with the patient briefly when serving the food tray.

h. Encourage family members to visit during mealtime. If present, a family member may want to feed the patient who needs assistance. Be sure that this is relaxing and safe for the patient.

i. When conditions allow for it, encourage the ambulatory patient to go to the dining hall for meals or open curtains in a double room so that patients may eat together. If the patient must eat alone, turn on the television or radio.

## 5-9. RESPONSIBILITIES OF THE PRACTICAL NURSE IN RELATION TO DIET THERAPY

a. The practical nurse should be familiar with the diet prescription and its therapeutic purpose. Although individual trays are carefully checked before leaving the Nutrition Care Division, mistakes can happen. Examine each tray with the patient's specific diet in mind. You should be able to recognize each type of diet.

b. You should relate the diet to body function and the condition being treated. For example, a low fat diet is usually the first step in treating patients with elevated blood lipids (hyperlipidemia). Hyperlipidemia may be caused by improper diet or it may have a secondary cause, such as hypothyroidism or renal failure. Untreated hyperlipidemia can lead to coronary heart disease.

c. Be able to explain the general principles of the diet to the patient, and obtain the patient's cooperation.

(1) For example, teach a diabetic patient the relationship between his insulin and the amount of food consumed.

(2) Observe the patient's reaction to the diet. If the patient understands the relationship between his condition and his diet, and is shown that he can continue to enjoy most of his favorite foods, he is more likely to remain on the diet.

d. Help plan for the patient's continued care.

(1) Most patients are hospitalized only during the acute and early convalescent phases of their illness so it may be necessary to continue a special diet at home.

(2) Chronic conditions, such as diabetes or hypertension, require permanent dietary alterations.

(3) Be aware of the patient's home situation and the problems that the diet may cause. The patient and his family will have to adjust their meal plans.

(4) Request a consultation for the patient with the dietitian early in the hospitalization to allow for instructions and follow-up care.

## 5-10. REASONS FOR THERAPEUTIC DIETS

Nutritional support is fundamental, whether the patient has an acute illness or faces chronic disease and its treatment. Frequently, it is the primary therapy in itself. The registered dietitian, along with the physician, carries the major responsibility for the patient's nutritional care. The nurse, and other primary care practitioners provide essential support. Valid nutritional care must be planned on identified personal needs and goals of the individual patient. We should not lose sight of the reasons for therapeutic diets.

a. **To Maintain or Improve Nutritional Status.** The stereotypical all-American family with two parents and two children eating three balanced meals each day with a ban on snacks is no longer a common reality. Widespread societal changes include an increase in the number of women in the work force and families who rely on food items and cooking methods that save time, space, and labor. The "snack" is clearly a significant component of foods consumed. A therapeutic diet may be planned to promote foods that contribute to nutritional adequacy.

b. **To Improve Nutritional Deficiencies.** Dietary surveys have shown that approximately one third of the US population lives on diets with less than the optimal amounts of various nutrients. Such nutritionally deficient persons are limited in physical work capacity, immune system function, and mental activity. They lack the nutritional reserves to meet any added physiologic or metabolic demands from injury or illness, or to sustain fetal development during pregnancy.

c. **To Maintain, Increase, or Decrease Body Weight.** Despite the growing interest in physical fitness, one out of every four Americans is on a weight reduction diet. Only 5 percent of these dieters manage to maintain their weight at the new lower level after such a diet. The basic cause is an underlying energy imbalance: more energy intake as food than energy output as basal metabolic needs and physical activity. Being underweight is a less common problem in the US. It is usually associated with poor living conditions or long-term disease. Resistance to infection is lowered and strength is reduced. Other causes for a person being underweight are self-imposed eating disorders, malabsorption resulting from a diseased gastrointestinal tract, hyperthyroidism, and increased physical activity without a corresponding increase in food intake.

d. **To Alleviate Stress to Certain Organs or to the Whole Body.**

(1) When loss of teeth or dental problems make chewing difficult, a dental soft diet may be used. All foods are soft-cooked, meats are ground and sometimes mixed with gravy or sauces.

(2) Peptic ulcer is the general term given to an eroded mucosal lesion in the central portion of the gastrointestinal tract. Little is understood about its underlying causes. The prime objective in medical management is to provide psychologic rest and support tissue healing. Three factors form the basis of care: drug therapy, rest, and diet. The bland diets used in the past for treatment of peptic ulcer have proved to be ineffective. Positive individual needs and a flexible program of a regular diet, including good food sources of dietary fiber, milk, and other protein foods prevail today.

(3) General functional disorders of the intestine may be caused by irritation of the mucous membrane. Symptoms vary between constipation and diarrhea. Dietary measures are designed to provide optimal nutrition and regulate bowel motility. There should be additional amounts of fruits, vegetables, and whole grains. The fiber content may need to be decreased during periods of diarrhea or excessive flatulence.

(4) Organic diseases of the intestine fall into three general groups: anatomic changes, malabsorption syndromes, and inflammatory bowel disease with infectious mucosal changes.

(a) Diverticulosis is an example of anatomic changes. Current studies and clinical practice have demonstrated that diverticular disease is better managed with a high-fiber diet than with restricted amounts of fiber used in former practices.

(b) Celiac disease is an example of malabsorption syndrome. Since the discovery that the gliadin fraction in gluten (a protein found mainly in wheat) is the causative factor, a low-gluten, gliadin-free diet has resulted in marked remission of symptoms.

(c) Inflammatory bowel disease is a term applied to both ulcerative colitis and Crohn's disease. These two diseases have similar clinical and pathologic features. They are particularly prevalent in industrialized areas of the world, suggesting that the environment plays a significant role. The two goals of a therapeutic diet are to support the tissue-healing process and prevent nutritional deficiency. The diet must supply about 100 grams of protein per day through elemental formulas or protein supplements with food as tolerated.

e. **To Eliminate Food Substances to Which the Patient may be Allergic.** There are three basic approaches to the diagnosis and treatment of food allergies: clinical assessment, laboratory tests, and dietary manipulation. Diet therapy is individualized.

f. **To Adjust Diet Composition.** A therapeutic diet may be ordered to aid digestion, metabolism, or excretion of certain nutrients or substances.

## 5-11. STANDARD HOSPITAL DIETS

The types of standard diets used by the Department of the Army are found in TM 8-500, Nutritional Support Handbook.

a. **Clear Liquid Diet.** This diet is indicated for the postoperative patient's first feeding when it is necessary to fully ascertain return of gastrointestinal function. It may also be used during periods of acute illness, in cases of food intolerance, and to reduce colon fecal matter for diagnostic procedures.

(1) The diet is limited to fat-free broth or bouillon, flavored gelatin, water, fruit drinks without pulp, fruit ice, Popsicles®, tea, coffee or coffee substitutes, and sugar. No cream or creamers are used. Carbonated beverages may be included when ordered by the physician; however, they are often contraindicated.

(2) The standard menu mat (DA Form 2902-15R) provides approximately 1146 calories. This diet is below the recommended dietary allowances (RDA) for all nutrients tabulated except for Vitamin C (ascorbic acid). If the patient is to be on clear liquids for an extended period of time, the portion sizes should be increased or an accepted enteral formula may be provided.

b. **Full Liquid Diet.** This diet is used when a patient is unable to chew or swallow solid food because of extensive oral surgery, facial injuries, esophageal strictures, and carcinomas of the mouth and esophagus. It may be used to transition between a clear liquid and a regular diet for the post-surgical patient.

(1) The diet consists of foods, which are liquid at room or body temperature, and will easily flow through a straw. Included in the full liquid diet are all juices, strained soups, thinned, cooked cereals, custards, ice cream, sherbet, and milk. A high protein beverage is given at breakfast and between meals. Commercially prepared liquid supplements may also be used.

(2) The standard menu mat (DA Form 2902-12-R) provides approximately 2777 calories. This diet is slightly below the RDA in iron for females, and in niacin for men.

c. **Advanced Full Liquid Diet.** This diet may be prescribed to meet the nutritive requirements of a patient who must receive a full liquid diet for an extended period of time or who has undergone oral surgery and must have foods, which can pass through a straw.

(1) The foods permitted are the same as those allowed on the full liquid diet. The advanced full liquid diet is made more nutritious by the addition of blended, thinned, and strained meat, potatoes, and vegetables. High-protein beverages are served with meals and between meals.

(2) The standard menu mat provides approximately 4028 calories. The advanced full liquid diet meets the RDA for all nutrients tabulated.

d. **Tonsillectomy and Adenoidectomy Cold Liquid Diet.** This diet is used following a tonsillectomy and adenoidectomy (T&A). It is also used when only fluids or soothing foods in liquid form are tolerated.

(1) The T&A cold liquid diet provides only cold liquids, which are free of irritants or acid properties. Foods allowed are flavored gelatins, ice cream, sherbet, and milk. A high protein beverage is served between meals.

(2) The standard menu mat is DA Form 2902-14-R. The T&A cold liquid diet does not meet the RDA for niacin and Vitamin A for adult males or children ages 4 to 10, and is below the RDA for thiamine for children ages 1 to 4. It does not meet the RDA for iron for any age group.

e. **Soft Diet.** The soft diet is prescribed for patients unable to tolerate a regular diet. It is part of the progressive stages of diet therapy after surgery or during recovery from an acute illness.

(1) The diet consists of solid foods that are prepared without added black pepper, chili powder, or chili pepper. It does <u>not</u> contain whole grain cereals or salads with raw, fresh fruits and vegetables. Serving sizes are small to provide a gradual increase in the amount of food from the liquid diet.

(2) The standard menu mat (DA Form 2902-4-R) provides approximately 2236 calories. This diet does not meet the RDA in iron for females or thiamine for males, nor niacin for either males or females.

f. **Dental Soft Diet.** This diet is prescribed for patients who are recovering from extensive oral surgery, have severe gingivitis, have had multiple extractions, have chewing difficulties because of tooth loss or other oral condition, or for the very elderly, toothless patient.

(1) The diet is composed of seasoned ground meats, vegetables, and other foods, which are easily chewed. The individuality of the patient must not be overlooked when a dental soft diet is prescribed. Many patients resent being served ground meat.

(2) Standard menu mats available are DA Form 2902-6-R (dental soft diet) and DA Form 2906-13-R (dental soft, 2000 mg sodium diet). The dental soft diet does not meet the RDA in thiamin for males, nor iron for females.

g. **Regular Diet.** Regular diets are planned to meet the nutritional needs of adolescents, adults, and geriatric phases of the life span.

(1) The regular diet includes the basic food groups and a variety of foods. The basic food groups include meat, milk, vegetables, fruits, bread and cereal, fats, and sweets.

(2) The standard menu mat, DA Form 2901-R (Regular Diet) provides approximately 3375 calories. The selective menu is developed by each individual hospital according to patient needs, food availability, and cost. The regular diet is designed to provide exceptionally generous amounts of all recognized nutrients and meets or exceeds the RDA for all nutrients tabulated.

(3) The Food Guide Pyramid is an outline of what we should eat each day (see figure 5-1). It shows six food groups, but emphasizes foods from the five food groups shown in the lower sections of the Pyramid. You need food from each group for good health. Each of the food groups provides some of the nutrients you need. Food from one group cannot replace those of another group.

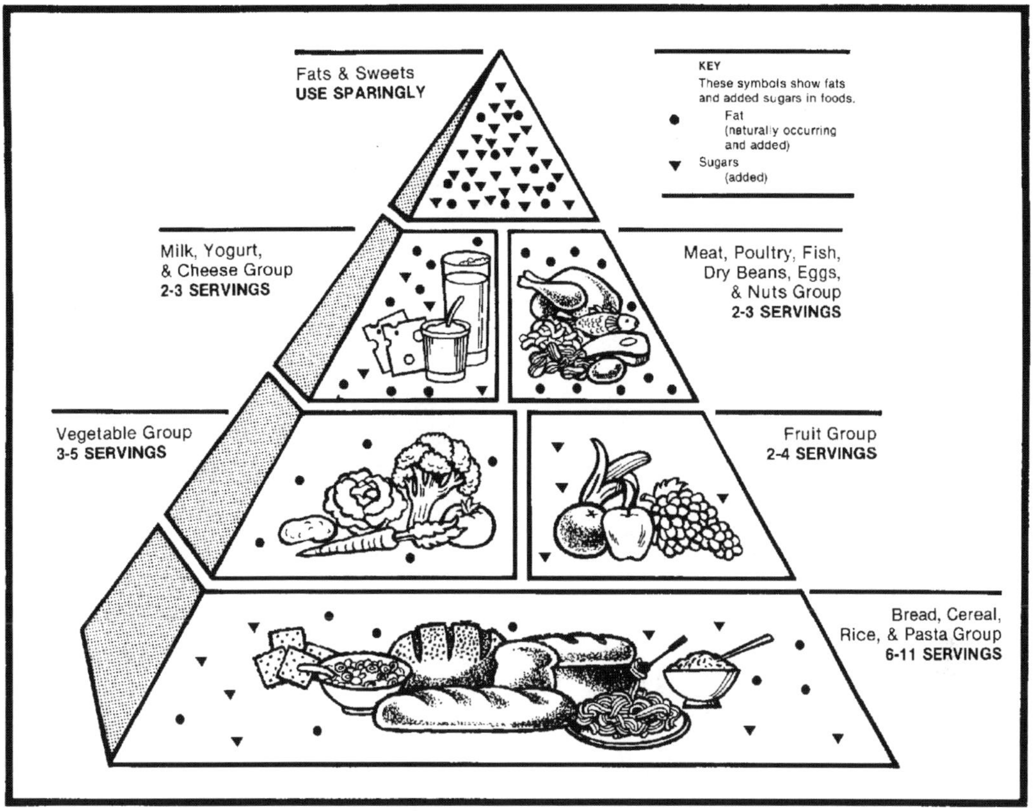


Figure 5-1. Food Guide Pyramid.

h. **Diabetic Diet.** The diabetic diet is indicated in the treatment of the metabolic disorder diabetes mellitus. This disease results from an inadequate production or utilization of insulin. The object of treating the diabetic patient by diet, with or without insulin or oral drugs, is to prevent hyperglycemia, hypoglycemia, glycosuria, and ketosis.

(1) The diabetic food exchange lists are the basis for a meal planning system that was designed by a committee of the American Diabetes Association and The American Dietetic Association. The system lists: meat exchange, bread exchange, fruit and juice exchange, vegetable exchange, milk exchange and fat exchange. The number of exchanges allowed is based upon the doctor's order and the dietitian's calculations. Each diabetic diet should be individualized to meet the needs of the patient. The foods in each exchange contain the same amount of calories, carbohydrate, protein, and fat per portion size. Patients select from the exchange based upon their preference.

(2) The adequacy and possible deficiencies depend on the calories. A diet of less than 1200 calories for women and less than 1500 calories for men would have a great chance of being deficient in some nutrients.

(3) The goals of the diabetic diet are:

(a) To improve the overall health of the patient by attaining and maintaining optimum nutrition.

(b) To attain and maintain an ideal body weight.

(c) To provide for the pregnant woman and her fetus: normal physical growth in the child, adequate nutrition for lactation needs if she chooses to breast-feed her infant.

(d) To maintain plasma glucose as near the normal physiologic range as possible.

(e) To prevent or delay the development and progression of cardiovascular, renal, retinal, neurologic, and other complications associated with diabetes.

(f) To modify the diet as necessary for complications of diabetes and for associated diseases.

i. **Liberal Bland Diet.** This diet is indicated for any medical condition requiring treatment for the reduction of gastric secretion, such as gastric or duodenal ulcers, gastritis, esophagitis, or hiatal hernia.

(1) The diet consists of any variety of regular foods and beverages, which are prepared or consumed without black pepper, chili powder, or chili pepper. Chocolate, coffee, tea, caffeine-containing products, and decaffeinated coffee are not included in the diet. The diet should be as liberal as possible and individualized to meet the needs of the patient. Foods, which cause the patient discomfort, should be avoided. Small, frequent feedings may be prescribed to lower the acidity of the gastric content and for the physical comfort of the patient.

(2) The standard menu mat, DA Form 2902-1-R, provides 3213 calories. The liberal bland diet is slightly below the RDA for thiamine and niacin for men 19 to 22 years of age. It is also below the RDA in iron for women of all ages.

j. **Low Fat Diet**. Fat restricted diets may be indicated in diseases of the liver, gallbladder, or pancreas in which disturbances of the digestion and absorption of fat may occur (pancreatitis, post-gastrointestinal surgery, cholelithiasis, and cystic fibrosis).

(1) The diet contains approximately 40 grams of fat from the six ounces of lean meat, fish, or poultry, one egg and three teaspoons of butter, margarine, or other allowed fats. Only lean, well-trimmed meats and skim milk are used. All foods are prepared without fat.

(2) The standard menu mat, DA Form 2905-R, provides approximately 2168 calories. Caloric content of the diet can be increased by adding allowable breads, vegetables, fruits, or skim milk. The diet is below the RDA in iron for males between the ages of 11 and 22 and females 11 through 50 years of age.

k. **Sodium Restricted Diet.** The purpose of the sodium-restricted diet is to promote loss of body fluids for patients who are unable to excrete the element normally because of a pathological condition. The diet is indicated for the prevention, control, and elimination of edema in congestive heart failure; cirrhosis of the liver with ascites; renal disease complicated by either edema or hypertension; when administration of adrenocorticotrophic hormone (ACTH) or steroids are prescribed, and for certain endocrine disorders such as Cushing's disease and hypothyroidism.

(1) The sodium-restricted diets provide a specific sodium level or a range of sodium. The diet order must indicate the specific sodium level or range desired either in milligrams (mg) or mill equivalent (mEq). Terms such as "salt free" and "low sodium" are not sufficient.

(a) All foods on the 500 mg and 1000 mg sodium diets are prepared without the addition of salt, and foods high in sodium are omitted. The 500 mg sodium diet uses both sodium restricted bread and margarine. The 1000 mg sodium diet uses sodium restricted margarine and regular bread. The 2000 mg sodium diet uses regular bread and margarine, and regular cereal and desserts prepared with sodium.

(b) The standard menu mats, DA Form 2906-1-R (500 mg sodium diet), DA Form 2906-2-R (1000 mg sodium diet), and DA Form 2906-3-R (2000 mg sodium diet), provide between 2083 and 2554 calories.

(2) The diets are below the RDA in iron for males ages 11 to 22 and for females ages 11 to 50. Thiamine is inadequate for males at all levels. Calcium and niacin are also low for certain diets and ages.

## 5-12. PREPARING THE PATIENT FOR MEALS

a. As a nurse, your duties may include serving the diet trays at mealtime. For many patients, mealtime is the high point of the day. The patients are more apt to have a better appetite, eat more, and enjoy their food more if you prepare them for their meals before the trays arrive.

(1) Provide for elimination by offering the bedpan or urinal or assisting the patient to the bathroom.

(2) Assist the patient to wash hands and face as needed.

(3) Create an attractive and pleasant environment for eating. Remove distracting articles such as an emesis basin or a urinal, and use a deodorizer to remove

unpleasant odors in the room. See that the room is well lighted and at a comfortable temperature.

(4) Position the patient for the meal. If allowed, elevate the head of the bed or assist the patient to sit up in a chair.

(5) Clear the overbed table to make room for the diet tray.

b. Avoid treatments such as enemas, dressings, and injections immediately before and after meals.

**5-13. CLOSING**

Helping patients meet their nutritional needs is a challenging task for a nurse. Ordering the tray and delivering it to the patient's bedside is not enough. You must see that he eats the food needed to meet his body requirements. Provide the patient with assistance to complete selective menus that meet his food preferences as much as possible. See to his comfort at mealtime. Without proper nutrition, the healing process slows down and the patient's condition does not improve as quickly as it should. You should always remember that the dietitians and hospital food service specialist (MOS 91M) of the hospital's Nutrition Care Division are available to you as experts in all aspects of patient nutrition care. Ask for their advice or intervention when you believe a patient's condition requires it.

***Continue with Exercises***

**EXERCISE, LESSON 5**

**INSTRUCTIONS:** To complete this exercise, circle the letter of the response that best answers the question or completes the statement or write the answer in the space provided. After you have completed the all of the exercises, turn to "Solutions to Exercises" at the end of this lesson and check your answers. If you have responded to any of the exercises incorrectly, reread the material referenced after the answer.

1. Six factors that influence eating patterns are:

   a. ______________________________.

   b. ______________________________.

   c. ______________________________.

   d. ______________________________.

   e. ______________________________.

   f. ______________________________.

2. List four factors that alter a hospitalized patient's eating patterns.

   a. ______________________________.

   b. ______________________________.

   c. ______________________________.

   d. ______________________________.

3. Certain factors in illness may alter food intake. List four of these factors.

   a. ______________________________.

   b. ______________________________.

   c. ______________________________.

   d. ______________________________.

4. List four reasons for hospitalized patients being at risk of malnutrition.

   a. ______________________________________________.

   b. ______________________________________________.

   c. ______________________________________________.

   d. ______________________________________________.

5. One nursing intervention, which may help the patient to meet his nutritional needs, is to inform the ________________ or the __________________________________ of any special needs that the patient may have.

6. In relation to diet therapy, responsibilities of the practical nurse are to:

   a. ______________________________________________.

   b. ______________________________________________.

   c. ______________________________________________.

   d. ______________________________________________.

7. Six reasons for therapeutic diets are:

   a. ______________________________________________.

   b. ______________________________________________.

   c. ______________________________________________.

   d. ______________________________________________.

   e. ______________________________________________.

   f. ______________________________________________.

8. The diet limited to fat-free broth or bouillon, flavored gelatin, water, fruit drinks without pulp, fruit ice, Popsicles®, tea, and coffee is the:

   a. Full liquid diet.

   b. T&A cold liquid diet.

   c. Clear liquid diet.

   d. Advanced full liquid diet.

9. The ____________________________ diet may be prescribed to meet the nutritive requirements of a patient who must receive a full liquid diet for an extended period of time or who must have foods which can pass through a straw.

10. The _____________________ diet consists of small serving sizes of solid foods, but does not contain whole grain cereals or salads with raw, fresh fruits and vegetables.

11. The diabetic ________________________________ are the basis for a meal planning system designed by a committee of The American Diabetes Association and The American Dietetic Association.

12. The diet composed of seasoned ground meats, vegetables, and other foods which are easily chewed is the:

   a. Soft diet.

   b. Bland diet.

   c. Dental soft diet.

   d. Liberal bland diet.

13. The ____________________________ is an outline of what we should eat each day. It shows _________________________________ food groups.

14. The sodium-restricted diet is indicated for:

    a. ______________________________________________________.

    b. ______________________________________________________.

    c. ______________________________________________________.

15. The diet order for a sodium-restricted diet must indicate the specific sodium level or range.

    a. True.

    b. False.

16. All foods on the 500 mg and 1000 mg sodium diets are prepared. ____________ __________________________. Foods ____________________________ are omitted.

17. Patients are more apt to have a better appetite, eat more, and enjoy their food more if you prepare them for their meals ____________________________________.

18. Immediately before and after meals, the nurse should avoid treatments such as _________________, __________________ and ______________________.

***Check Your Answers on Next Page***

**SOLUTIONS TO EXERCISE, LESSON 5**

1. Social aspects.
   Emotional aspects.
   Food fads and fallacies.
   Financial considerations.
   Physical condition.
   Cultural heritage/religion. (paras 5-2a--f)

2. The forced menu of available foods.
   The forced eating schedule.
   Isolation from family and significant others.
   Restriction in activity. (paras 5-5a--d)

3. Any **four** of the following are correct.
   The disease process.
   Drug therapy.
   Anxiety about his/her illness.
   Diet restrictions.
   Changes in usual activity level.
   Loneliness. (paras 5-6a--f)

4. The effect of the disease on metabolism.
   The disease may cause problems with absorption.
   Treatment may cause problems with intake, digestion, or absorption.
   Anxiety and stress may reduce the patient's appetite. (paras 5-7a--d)

5. Dietitian; hospital food service specialist. (para 5-8f)

6. Be familiar with the diet prescription and its therapeutic purpose.
   Relate the diet to body function and the condition being treated.
   Be able to explain the general principles of the diet to the patient.
   Help plan for the patient's continued care. (paras 5-9a--d)

7. To maintain or improve nutritional status.
   To improve nutritional deficiencies.
   To maintain, increase, or decrease body weight.
   To alleviate stress to certain organs or to the whole body.
   To eliminate food substances to which the patient may be allergic.
   To adjust diet composition in order to aid digestion, metabolism, or excretion of certain nutrients or substances. (paras 5-10a--e)

8. c (para 5-11a(1))

9. Advanced full liquid. (para 5-11c)

10. Soft. (para 5-11e(1))

11. Exchange lists. (para 5-11h(1))

12. c (para 5-11f(1))

13. Food Guide Pyramid; six. (para 5-11g(3))

14. Prevention, control, and elimination of edema in congestive heart failure.
    Cirrhosis of the liver with ascites.
    Renal disease complicated by either edema or hypertension. (para 5-11k)

15. a (para 5-11k(1))

16. Without the addition of salt; high in sodium. (para 5-11k(1)(a))

17. Before the trays arrive. (para 5-12a)

18. Enemas, dressings, injections. (para 5-12b)

***End of Lesson 5***

## LESSON ASSIGNMENT

**LESSON 6** Introduction to Physical Assessment

**TEXT ASSIGNMENT** Paragraphs 6-1 through 6-9

**LESSON OBJECTIVES** After completing this lesson, you should be able to:

6-1. Define physical assessment.

6-2. Select the purposes for performing a physical assessment.

6-3. Select the nursing considerations for preparing a patient for a physical assessment.

6-4. Identify the basic techniques used in performing a physical assessment.

6-5. Select the specific areas assessed when performing a general appearance and behavioral assessment.

6-6. Identify the components of a systemic, head-to-toe physical assessment.

6-7. Select the medical terminology related to physical assessment when given the definition.

6-8. Identify guidelines for documentation of the physical assessment.

**SUGGESTION** After studying the assignment, complete the exercises at the end of this lesson. These exercises will help you to achieve the lesson objectives.

## LESSON 6

## INTRODUCTION TO PHYSICAL ASSESSMENT

### 6-1. INTRODUCTION

An accurate physical assessment requires an organized and systematic approach using the techniques of inspection, palpation, percussion, and auscultation. It also requires a trusting relationship and rapport between the nurse and the patient to decrease the stress the patient may have from being physically exposed and vulnerable. The patient will be much more relaxed and cooperative if you explain what will be done and the reason for doing it. While the findings of a nursing assessment do sometimes contribute to the identification of a medical diagnosis, the unique focus of a nursing assessment is on the patient's responses to actual or potential problems.

### 6-2. FACTS ABOUT PHYSICAL ASSESSMENT

a. Physical assessment is an organized systemic process of collecting objective data based upon a health history and head-to-toe or general systems examination. A physical assessment should be adjusted to the patient, based on his needs. It can be a complete physical assessment, an assessment of a body system, or an assessment of a body part.

b. The physical assessment is the first step in the nursing process. It provides the foundation for the nursing care plan in which your observations play an integral part in the assessment, intervention, and evaluation phases.

c. The chances of overlooking important data are greatly reduced because the physical assessment is performed in an organized, systematic manner, instead of a random manner.

### 6-3. PURPOSES OF A PHYSICAL ASSESSMENT

a. A comprehensive patient assessment yields both subjective and objective findings. Subjective findings are obtained from the health history and body systems review. Objective findings are collected from the physical examination.

(1) Subjective data are apparent only to the person affected and can be described or verified only by that person. Pain, itching, and worrying are examples of subjective data.

(2) Objective data are detectable by an observer or can be tested by using an accepted standard. A blood pressure reading, discoloration of the skin, and seeing the patient in the act of crying are examples of objective data.

(3) Objective data are sometimes called ***signs***, and subjective data are sometimes called ***symptoms***.

(4) ***Data*** means more than signs or symptoms; it also includes *demographics*, or patient information that is not related to a disease process.

b. The purposes for a physical assessment are:

(1) To obtain baseline physical and mental data on the patient.

(2) To supplement, confirm, or question data obtained in the nursing history.

(3) To obtain data that will help the nurse establish nursing diagnoses and plan patient care.

(4) To evaluate the appropriateness of the nursing interventions in resolving the patient's identified pathophysiology problems.

## 6-4. CONSIDERATIONS IN PREPARING A PATIENT FOR A PHYSICAL ASSESSMENT

a. **Establish a Positive Nurse/Patient Rapport.** This relationship will decrease the stress the patient may have in anticipation of what is about to be done to him.

b. **Explain the Purpose for the Physical Assessment.** The purpose of the nursing assessment is to gather information about the patient's health so that you can plan individualized care for that patient. All other steps in the nursing process depend on the collection of relevant, descriptive data. The data must be factual, not interpretive.

c. **Obtain an Informed, Verbal Consent for the Assessment.** The chief source of data is usually the patient unless the patient is too ill, too young, or too confused to communicate clearly. Patients often appreciate detailed concern for their problems and may even enjoy the attention they receive.

d. **Ensure Confidentiality of All Data.** If possible, choose a private place where others cannot overhear or see the patient. Explain what information is needed and how it will be used. It is also important to convey where the data will be recorded and who will see it. In some situations, you should explain to the patient his rights to privileged communication with health care providers.

e. **Provide Privacy From Unnecessary Exposure.** Assure as much privacy as possible by using drapes appropriately and closing doors.

f. **Communicate Special Instructions to the Patient.** As you proceed with the examination, inform the patient of what you intend to do and how he can help, especially when you anticipate possible embarrassment or discomfort.

## 6-5. BASIC TECHNIQUES USED IN PERFORMING A PHYSICAL ASSESSMENT

a. **Inspection.** Visual examination of a person is called inspection. This is done in an orderly manner, focusing on one area of the body at a time.

b. **Palpation.** Examination by touch is called palpation (figure 6-1). The nurses feels for texture, size, consistency, and location of body parts.

c. **Auscultation.** Examination by listening for sounds produced within the body is called auscultation. The sounds most frequently listened for are those of the abdominal and thoracic viscera and the movement of blood in the cardiovascular system. Direct auscultation, using the ear only, is seldom done. Indirect auscultation is generally carried out with a stethoscope.

d. **Percussion.** Examination of the body by tapping it with the fingers is called percussion (figure 6-2). Percussion is a special assessment skill that the practical nurse is not required to perform. This technique is usually performed by a registered nurse (RN) or a physician.

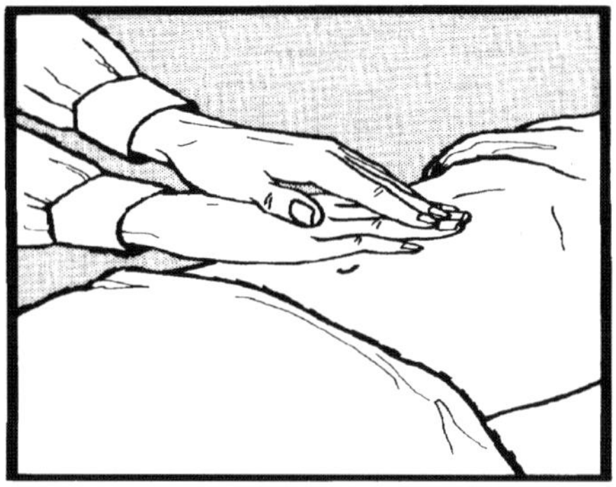

Figure 6-1. Palpation.

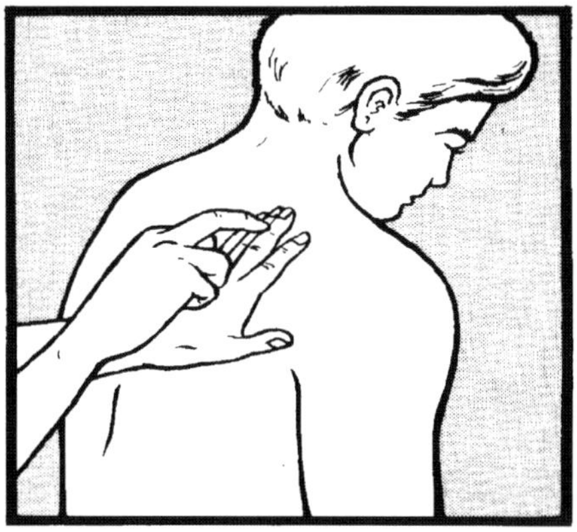

Figure 6-2. Percussion.

## 6-6. AREAS OF GENERAL APPEARANCE AND BEHAVIORAL ASSESSMENT

a. **Demographic Data.** You begin the assessment by collecting personal information, which includes name, age, sex, marital status, race, and religion. This identifies the patient and provides important demographic data.

b. **Body Build.** Observe the patient's general appearance and health state in relation to his age and lifestyle. Determine the patient's height, weight, and vital signs at this time.

c. **Posture and Gait**. Observe whether the patient is erect or slouched, steady or unsteady. Posture can indicate mood. For example, a slumped position may reflect depression; too rigid and upright a position may indicate anxiety.

d. **Hygiene and Grooming.** Look for cleanliness of nails, hair, skin, and overall appearance. Usually, you can assess these gradually while observing other parts of the body for data. Observe the skin for color, texture, temperature, and lesions. Lesions warrant particular attention during assessment. Some primary skin lesions are:

(1) Nodule--a solid mass extending into the dermis.

(2) Tumor--a solid mass larger than a nodule.

(3) Cyst--an encapsulated fluid-filled mass in the dermis or subcutaneous layer.

(4) Wheal--a relatively reddened, flat, localized collection of fluid. An example is hives.

(5) Vesicle--circumscribed elevation containing serous fluid or blood. An example is chickenpox.

(6) Bulla-- large fluid-filled vesicle. An example is a second-degree burn.

(7) Pustule--a vesicle or bulla filled with pus. An example is acne.

e. **Dress.** Observe the patient's clothing in relation to age, climate, socioeconomic status, and culture. Notice whether the clothing is clean, properly buttoned, or zipped. The patient's dress may reflect the cold intolerance of hypothyroidism. Slippers or untied shoelaces suggest edema.

f. **Body and Breath Odors.** Malodorous body or breath may indicate pulmonary infections, uremia, or liver failure. A breath odor of acetone may be due to diabetes. Although odors give important clues, avoid the common mistake of assuming that alcohol on a patient's breath explains neurologic or mental status findings. Alcoholic breath does not necessarily mean alcoholism.

g. **Attitude.** The patient's attitude is reflected in his appearance, speech, and behavior. The patient may be aloof and unwilling to participate in the interview. He may verbalize anger or fear. Some patients have a "take care of me" attitude and expect nurses and other health care personnel to magically know everything about them. Such findings should be noted as part of your general impression.

h. **Affect/Mood.** Affect is the emotional state as it appears to others. Mood is the emotional state as described by the patient. Observe the patient's facial expression. No part of the body is as expressive as the face. Feelings of joy, sadness, fear, surprise, anger, and disgust are conveyed by facial expression. Facial expressions generally are not consciously controlled.

i. **Speech.** Assess the patient's speech for loudness, clarity, pace, and coherence. Observe the patient for poor articulation of words and language difficulty. Patients who are not fluent in English or have limited education are sometimes mistakenly labeled as "indifferent" or "noncommunicative."

## 6-7. COMPONENTS OF A PHYSICAL ASSESSMENT

a. **Health History.** During this assessment step, you interview the patient to obtain a history so that the nursing care plan may be patterned to meet the patient's individual needs. The history should clearly identify the patient's strengths and weaknesses, health risks such as hereditary and environmental factors, and potential and existing health problems. Both the seating arrangement and the distance from the patient are important in establishing a relaxed and comfortable environment for data collection. Chairs placed at right angles to each other about 3 feet apart facilitate an easy exchange of information. If the patient is in bed, be seated in a chair at a 45-degree angle to the bed. If possible, communicate with the patient at eye level. State your name and status and the purpose of the interview. During the introduction, assess the patient's comfort and ability to participate in the interview. Terminate the interview when you have obtained the data you need or the patient cannot provide more information. You need the following information in order to form the subjective database.

(1) <u>Chief complaint</u>. Record the chief complaint as a brief statement of whatever is troubling the patient and the duration of time the problem has existed. The chief complaint is the signs and symptoms causing the patient to seek medical attention. Generally, it is the answer to the question, "What brought you into the hospital (or clinic) today?" If a well person is seeking a routine physical, there is no actual chief complaint. Record his reason for the visit and the date of his last contact with a medical treatment facility.

(2) <u>Past medical history</u>. This provides background for understanding the patient as a whole and his present illness. It includes childhood illnesses, immunizations, allergies, hospitalizations and serious illnesses, accidents and injuries, medications, and habits.

(3) Family health history. This enhances your understanding of the environment in which the patient lives. Obtaining this information identifies genetic problems, communicable diseases, environmental problems, and interpersonal relationships. Specific inquiry should be made regarding the general state of health of parents, grandparents, siblings, spouse, and children. Record if the patient is adopted and has no access to his biological family's history.

b. **Vital Signs.** The patient's vital signs are part of the objective data that helps to better define the patient's condition and helps you in planning care. The following vital signs may be taken at the time the patient's height and weight are obtained.

(1) Blood pressure. Blood pressure may be taken in both arms. Record whether the patient was lying, sitting, or standing at the time the reading was obtained.

(2) Temperature. Record the temperature and whether it is an oral, axillary, or rectal temperature.

(3) Pulse. Peripheral pulses are graded on a scale of 0-4 by the following system.

(a) 0 = absent, without a pulse.

(b) +1 = diminished, barely palpable.

(c) +2 = average, slightly weak, but palpable.

(d) +3 = full and brisk, easily palpable.

(e) +4 = bounding pulse, sometimes visible.

c. **Head, Eyes, Ears, Nose, and Throat.** Assessment of the head begins with a general inspection. Continue the assessment by examining the eyes, ears, nose, and throat. Knowledge of the anatomy of the skull (figure 6-3) is helpful in localizing and describing physical findings.

(1) Observe the general size of the head. Inspect the skull for shape and symmetry. Note any deformities. Become familiar with the irregularities in a normal skull, such as those near the suture lines between the parietal and occipital bones. Part the hair in several places and inspect the scalp for scaliness, lumps, or other lesions. Note the quantity, distribution, pattern of loss if any, and texture of the hair. Observe the patient's facial expression and contours for asymmetry, involuntary movements, edema, and masses. Note the color, pigmentation, texture, and any lesions of the skin.

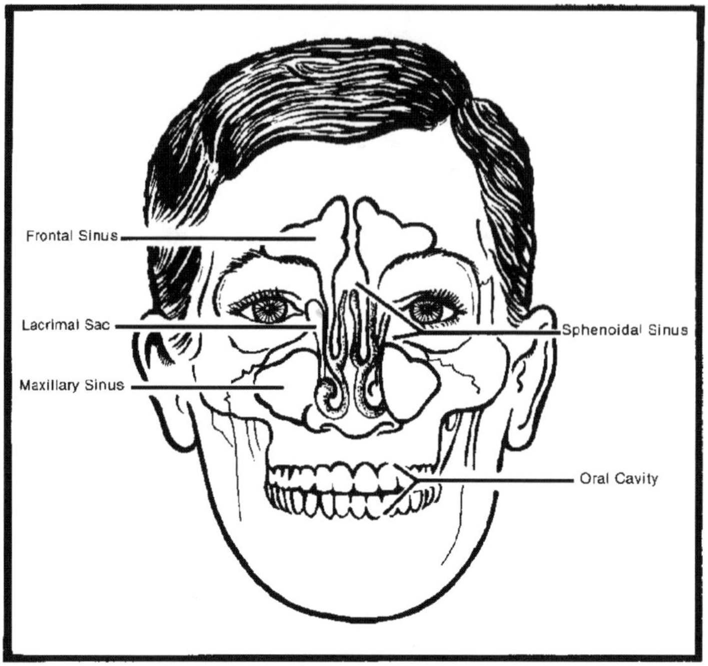


Figure 6-3. Anatomy of the skull.

(2) Inspect the eyes for symmetry, movement, and the condition of the pupils, iris, and sclera. Ask the patient to look up as you depress both lower lids with your thumbs, exposing the sclera and palpebral conjunctiva (lining of inner surface of the eyelids). See figure 6-4. Note the color and vascular pattern against the white background of the sclera. An apparently yellow sclera indicates jaundice. Pale palpebral conjunctiva may indicate anemia. Look for nodules or swelling. The pupils and iris are assessed together. Examine the pupils for color, shape, equality, reaction to light, and accommodation. The pupils are normally black in color, round, and equal. If the pupil

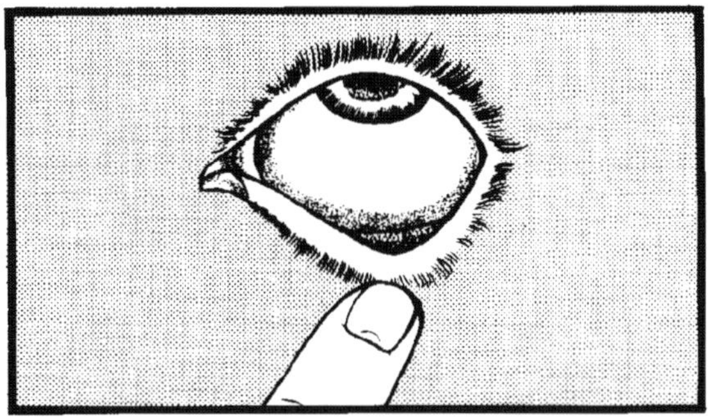

Figure 6-4. Exposing sclera and conjuctiva.

appears cloudy or discolored, the probable cause is a cataract. Health of the iris is determined by noting the regularity of the pupil. An irregular, constricted appearance to the pupil may result from edema due to inflammation of the iris. Screen visual acuity with any available print. If the patient cannot read the largest print, test the patient's ability to count your upraised fingers and distinguish light (such as your flashlight) from dark.

(3) The ear has three compartments: the external ear, the middle ear and the inner ear. Much of the middle ear and all of the inner ear are inaccessible to direct examination. The external ear is comprised of the auricle and ear canal. The ear canal opens behind the tragus. Assess the ears for hearing, symmetry, discharge, tinnitus (ringing in the ears), and vertigo (dizziness). Inspect each auricle of the ear and surrounding tissue for deformities, lumps, or skin lesions. If ear pain, discharge, or inflammation is present, move the auricle up and down, press the tragus, and press firmly just behind the ear. Movement of the auricle and tragus (figure 6-5) is painful in acute external otitis, but not in otitis media. Tenderness behind the ear may be present in otitis media. To estimate hearing, test one ear at a time. Ask the patient to occlude one ear with a finger. Stand 1 or 2 feet away, and whisper softly to the enucleated ear. Speak words with equally accented syllables, such as "homerun" or "four-nine." Make sure that the patient does not read your lips. Ask him to repeat what you have said.

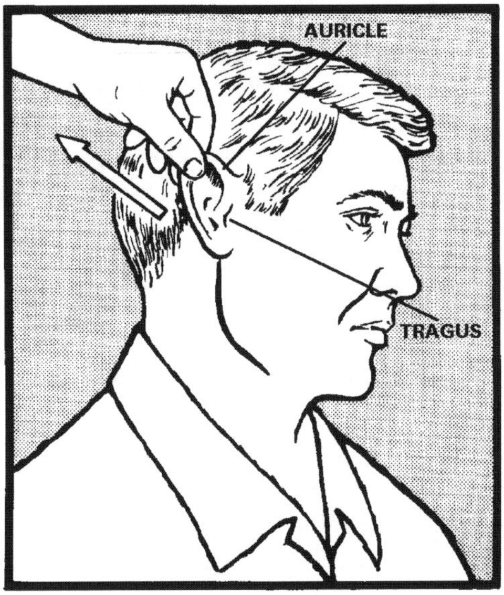


Figure 6-5. Movement of the auricle.

(4) The nose has two major functions. It enables us to use our sense of smell and it is the air conditioner of the respiratory system. Assess the nose for bone alignment and epistaxis (nosebleeds). Inspect the nasal mucosa and septum. If the patient complains of nosebleeds, ask him about the frequency, amount, and color of the nosebleeds. Inspect and palpate the outside of the nose. By using a penlight or

otoscope, you can get a partial view of each nasal vestibule. Note unusual skin markings, obvious deviation of the septum (asymmetry), discharge, or flaring of the nares. If the patient has a history of trauma to the nose, ask if there has been a change in his ability to smell. The nose, in conjunction with the paranasal sinuses, filters, warms, and moistens the air. The paranasal sinuses are air-filled cavities with ciliated mucous membrane linings. Only the frontal and maxillary sinuses are accessible to physical examination.

(5) Examine the throat. Include the lips, teeth, gums, tongue, buccal mucosa, uvula, and tonsils (figure 6-6). Observe the color and moisture of the lips. Note any cracking, lumps, or ulcers. Look into the patient's open mouth. Use a tongue blade and light to inspect the buccal mucosa for color, pigmentation, ulcers, white patches, and nodules. Patchy brown pigmentation is normal in black people. If the patient wears dentures, offer a container or paper towel and ask the patient to remove them so that you can look at the mucosa underneath. Look for swelling, bleeding, retraction, discoloration, and inflammation of the gums. Look for loose, missing, or carious teeth. Note abnormalities in the position or shape of the teeth. Inspect the back, sides, and undersurface of the tongue. Explain what you plan to do and put on gloves. Ask the patient to stick out his tongue. With one hand, grasp the tip of the tongue with a square of gauze and gently pull it to the side. Inspect the side of the tongue, and then palpate it with your other gloved hand, feeling for any hardening of tissue. Reverse the procedure for the other side of the tongue. With the patient's mouth still open, press the tongue blade down upon the midpoint of the arched tongue and inspect the uvula and tonsils. Note any evidence of pus, swelling, ulceration, or tonsillar enlargement. Whitish spots of normal tissue may sometimes be seen on the tonsils. White patches with redness and swelling, however, suggest pharyngitis. Break and discard the tongue blade after use. Inspect the neck, noting its symmetry and any masses or scars. Look for enlargement of the parotid or submaxillary glands, and note any visible lymph nodes.

**NOTE**: Determine the last medical check-up in each of these areas and the patient's need for corrective devices such as glasses, hearing aid, or braces.

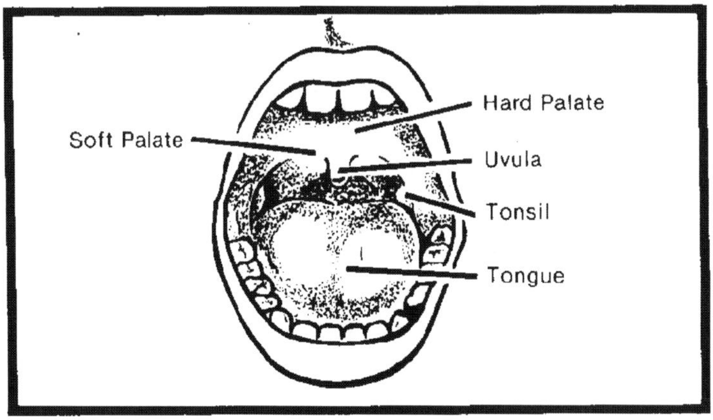


Figure 6-6. Oral cavity.

d. **Neurological Assessment.** There are two approaches to assessment of the neurologic system, depending on the condition of the patient and his chief complaint. If the patient is undergoing a routine health assessment, a screening level exam is appropriate. If the patient's chief complaint relates to the neurologic system, a more detailed assessment is required. A most important consideration is the cooperation and participation of the patient. The following assessments should be made.

(1) Mental status. Assess the patients level of consciousness and orientation to time, place, and person. Much of the mental status exam can be done during the interview. The patient's orientation to person, place, and time are intact if he knows who he is, where he is, and the time of day. Altered states of consciousness are:

(a) Conscious--Alert, awake, aware of one's self and environment.

(b) Confusion--Disorientation in time. Irritability and/or drowsiness. Misjudgment of sensory input. Shortened attention span. Decrease in memory.

(c) Delirium--Disorientation, fear. Misperception of sensory stimuli. Visual and auditory hallucinations. Loss of contact with environment.

(d) Stupor--Unresponsive, but can be aroused back to a near normal state.

(e) Coma--Unresponsive to external stimuli.

(f) Akinetic mutism--Alert-appearing, immobile. Mental activity absent.

(g) Locked-syndrome--No effective verbal or motor communication. Consciousness may be intact. EEG indicates a preservation of cerebral activity.

(h) Chronic vegetative state - Vital functions preserved with no evidence of active mental processes. EEG indicates absence of cerebral activity.

(2) Pupillary reaction. Examine the pupils for briskness, symmetry, and accommodation. Pupils are normally round and can range in size from "pinpoint" to occupying the entire space of the iris. Pupils normally constrict with increasing light and accommodation (ability of the lens to adjust to objects at varying distances).

(3) Strength. Muscle strength is tested against the resistance of the examiner. Strength will vary from person to person. Symmetrical responses are significant and permit you to use the patient as his own control. Assess strength in all extremities, the neck, and back.

(a) To assess strength in the upper extremities, have the patient squeeze your first two fingers with both hands. The grip should be reasonably strong, but most important; it should be equal in both hands. Apply resistance when the patient flexes the wrist and elbow. Note any pain or weakness the patient has.

(b) To assess shoulder and scapulae resistance, ask the patient to extend both arms out in front of him and resist the push that you will apply. Try to push the patient's arms down. This is a common site for sports injuries, arthritis, and bursitis. Ask the patient to raise both arms above his shoulders. Try to push his arms down to his sides. Instruct the patient to resist your efforts.

(c) Assess the lower extremities in a similar manner with the patient lying down. Ask the patient to raise his leg against your hand, which is applying pressure on the thigh, trying to flatten the leg. Ask the patient to flex his knees so that his feet are flat on the table. Place your hands laterally at both knees. Note any pain with this movement.

(4) Sensation. The sensory functions include touch, pain, vibration, position, temperature, and discrimination. If the patient complains of numbness, peculiar sensations, or paralysis, sensation should be checked more carefully over flexor and extensor surfaces of the extremities. Generally the face, arms, legs, hands, and feet are tested for touch and pain.

(a) Touch is tested with a wisp of cotton. Ask the patient to close his eyes and respond whenever the cotton touches his skin. Compare the sensation in symmetrical areas of the body, such as the cheeks.

(b) Test the sharpness or dullness of pain by using the pointed and the blunt end of a safety pin. Ask the patient to close his eyes and identify which end of the pin is touching him. Compare distal and proximal areas and note any areas of reduced or heightened sensations.

(c) The sense of vibration is tested with a tuning fork held firmly against a bone. Bones commonly used are located at the thumb side of the wrist, the outside of the elbow, either side of the ankle, and the knee. Test the distal bones of an extremity first. Strike the tuning fork fairly hard and hold it against the patient's skin. The patient should feel the vibration or buzz.

(d) The middle finger and large toe are used to test the sense of position. Ask the patient to close his eyes. While supporting the patient's arm with one hand, grasp the patient's middle finger firmly between the thumb and index finger of your other hand. Exert the same pressure on both sides of the patient's finger while moving it. To test the sense of position using the large toe, place the patient's heels on the examining table and grasp the toe in the same manner. Use a series of brisk up, down, and straight out movements before coming to rest in one of the three positions. Ask the patient to identify the position.

(e) Temperature sensation is determined by touching the patient's skin with tubes filled with hot and cold water. Ask the patient to identify which tube feels hot and which feels cold. This test is unnecessary if the "sensation of pain" test is normal.

(f) The ability to discriminate can be tested several ways. One way is *stereognosis* (the ability to recognize objects by touching them). Place small, familiar objects such as a coin, paper clip, or key in the patient's hand and ask him to identify it. Another way is the one- and two-point stimuli. Alternate touching the patient's fingertip with two pinpoints simultaneously and then with one pin. Have the patient discriminate between the one- and two-point stimuli.

e. **Respiration.** Respiration is assessed using inspection, palpation, and auscultation. Have the patient remove all clothing to the waist and assume a sitting position. Inspect the chest for posture, shape, and symmetry of expansion. Warm the diaphragm of the stethoscope in the palms of your hands and place it firmly against the patient's chest wall. Ask the patient to breath quietly with the mouth open.

(1) There are three types of normal breath sounds: vesicular, bronchial, and bronchovesicular. Vesicular sounds are soft, like a quiet rustle or swish. Bronchial sounds are loud, harsh, hollow blowing sounds usually heard over the trachea and major bronchi. Bronchial sounds are louder during expiration. Bronchovesicular sounds are a combination of the other two and are heard in the upper anterior chest on each side of the sternum and posteriorly between the scapulae. Deep breathing converts vesicular sounds into bronchovesicular sounds.

(2) Assess the respirations for rhythm. Note whether the patient's breathing is regular, irregular, labored, or non-labored.

(3) Respiratory rate is the number of breaths in one minute. Bradypnea is less than 10 breaths per minute. Dyspnea is difficult or painful breathing. Orthopnea is difficult breathing except in an upright position.

(4) Lung sounds include breath sounds, voice sounds, and abnormal sounds. Assess lung sounds by auscultation, using a stethoscope. Auscultate the anterior and posterior upper, middle and lower lobes. Rales are crackling, tinkling sounds that occur when fluid or secretions are trapped in the smaller bronchioles or alveoli. Rhonchi are the rumbling, rattling, or snoring sounds due to mucous and secretions in the bronchial tree. A wheeze is the raspy whistling or high-pitched sound that occurs as air moves through a constricted or obstructed passage in the upper airway or bronchioles.

(5) Note whether the patient has a cough and whether it is persistent, occasional, productive or nonproductive. If the cough is productive, note the amount and character of the secretions.

f. **Cardiovascular Assessment.** Palpation and auscultation are used in assessment of the cardiovascular system, which includes blood pressure, peripheral pulses, heart sounds, and circulatory perfusion. The patient's blood pressure is usually taken at the onset of the assessment and the pulses are palpated while the skin is being examined.

(1) To obtain an accurate blood pressure reading, you will need a stethoscope, a blood pressure cuff, and a sphygmomanometer. Be sure that the patient is relaxed and use a cuff that is not more than 20 percent wider than the diameter of the patient's limb and long enough to completely encircle it. If the patient is very obese, it may be necessary to use a thigh cuff on his arm. If possible, take the blood pressure in two positions, supine or seated and standing. Wrap the cuff around the arm so that it is about one inch above the bend of the elbow. Palpate the brachial artery and place the diaphragm of the stethoscope over the artery below, but not underneath, the cuff. Inflate the cuff 30 to 40°mm°Hg above the point at which the last sound is heard. Release the pressure slowly. Observe the pressure readings on the manometer and relate these to the sounds heard through the stethoscope. The systolic pressure is the point where the first tapping sound is heard. The diastolic pressure is the point where the sound disappears.

(2) Take the peripheral pulses with the patient in the supine position, using your index and middle finger. Palpate the apical, radial, dorsalis pedis, and posterior tibial pulses. The posterior tibial pulse is palpable behind and below the protuberance on the inside of the ankle. See figure 4-2 for arterial pulse sites.

(3) Several heart sounds can be heard by auscultation (see figure 6-7). The first two heart sounds are produced by closure of the valves of the heart. The first heart sound (S1) occurs when the ventricles have been sufficiently filled and the right and left atrioventricular (A-V) valves close. S1 is heard as one dull, low-pitched sound. After the ventricles empty their blood into the aorta and pulmonary arteries, the semilunar valves close, producing the second heart sound (S2). The second heart sound is shorter and has a higher pitch than S1. The two sounds occur within one second or less, depending on the heart rate. Systole is the period in which the ventricles are contracted. It begins with the first heart sound and ends at the second heart sound. Diastole is the period in which the ventricles are relaxed. Normally no sounds are heard during this period. The two heart sounds are audible anywhere in the region over the heart, but are best heard over specific valve areas. Rhythm is the pattern of the heartbeats and the intervals between the beats. It may be regular or irregular. Normally, equal time elapses between heartbeats. Any deviation from the normal pattern is ***arrhythmia***. Murmurs, produced by turbulent blood flow, may occur at any cardiac auscultation site. The volume of blood flow, the force of the contraction, and the degree of valve compromise all contribute to murmur quality. Descriptive terms are used to give the murmur character. Murmurs are "whooshing" sounds. Although the mitral sound is usually loudest, a stenotic mitral valve that moves very little may produce a muffled sound.

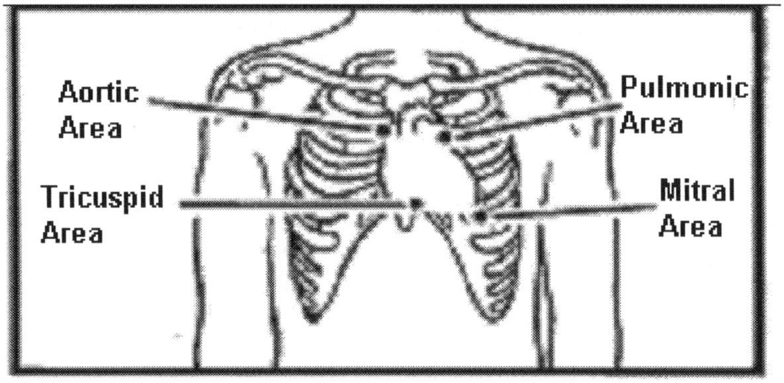


Figure 6-7. Areas to auscultate for heart sounds.

**Transmission of sounds with the closure of the heart valves.**

**A = Aortic**
**P = Pulmonic**
**T = Tricuspid**
**M = Mitral**

(4) Circulatory perfusion is blood flow through the vessels of a specific organ or tissue. Arteries carry blood away from the heart, the capillaries serve as in-between channels, and the veins carry blood toward the heart. Close examination of the extremities will indicate the quality of the arterial and venous systems. Capillaries are the smallest blood vessels. It is through their walls that oxygen and food are supplied to the individual cells. To test capillary refill to extremities, press on a toe or fingertip, observe blanching and the time it takes the area to return to its original color. Document the time in seconds.

g. **Gastrointestinal Assessment**. Inspection, palpation, and auscultation are used in gastrointestinal (GI) assessment. The GI system comprises two major components: the alimentary canal and the accessory organs. The alimentary canal includes the pharynx, esophagus, stomach, small intestine, and large intestine. Accessory organs aiding GI function include the salivary glands, liver, gallbladder and bile ducts, and the pancreas. Assessment of the gastrointestinal system includes inspection of the oral cavity (during HEENT evaluation), auscultation and palpation of the abdomen, and examination of the rectum.

(1) To ensure accurate abdominal assessment and consistent documentation of your findings, mentally divide the patient's abdomen into four quadrants (figure 6-8). Begin by inspecting the patient's entire abdomen, noting overall contour (flat, round, concave, protruding), skin integrity, appearance of the umbilicus, and any visible pulsations. Note any localized distention or irregular contours, rashes, dilated veins, and scars.

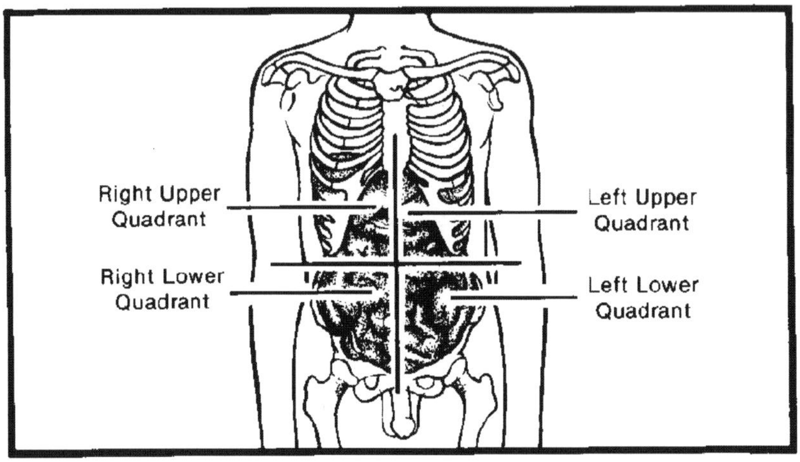


Figure 6-8. Abdominal regions.

(2) After inspecting the patient's abdomen, use a stethoscope to auscultate for bowel and vascular sounds. Lightly press the stethoscope diaphragm on the abdominal skin in all four quadrants. The bowel may be active, hyperactive, or hypoactive. Normally, air and fluid moving through the bowel by peristalsis create soft, bubbling sounds, mixed with clicks and gurgles, every 5 to 20 seconds. Loud, gurgling irregular sounds heard about every three seconds are hyperactive and may occur normally in a hungry person. Following, or when the colon is filled with feces, hypoactive bowel sounds may occur at a rate of one every minute or longer. Abdominal auscultation should be performed before percussion and palpation, because intestinal activity and bowel sounds may be altered by the motion of percussion and palpation.

(3) Palpation elicits useful clues about the character of the abdominal wall; the size, condition, and consistency of abdominal organs; the presence and nature of abdominal masses; and the presence, degree, and location of any abdominal pain. Gently press your fingertips about ½ inch into the abdominal wall. Move your hands in a slightly circular fashion so that the abdominal wall moves over the underlying structures. Note the character of the abdomen (soft, rigid, firm, tender, or nontender). Assess for organ location, masses, and areas of tenderness or increased muscle resistance. If you detect a mass, note its location, size, shape, degree of tenderness and mobility, and the presence of pulsations. When assessing a patient with abdominal pain, always auscultate and palpate in the painful quadrant last, touching the painful area may cause the patient to tense the abdominal muscles, making further assessment difficult.

**NOTE:** Do not palpate a pulsating midline mass; it may be a dissecting aneurysm, which can rupture under the pressure of palpation. Report the mass to a doctor.

(4) Gather information about the patient's appetite during the interview. Ask the patient if he has lost weight.

(5) Gather information about the patient's elimination patterns and the character of his stools. Ask the patient when he had his last bowel movement and if he has nausea, vomiting, diarrhea, or constipation.

(6) A routine rectal examination is performed if the patient is over age 40, if the patient has a history of bowel elimination changes or anal discomfort, and for an adult male with a urinary problem.

(7) If the patient is ambulatory, ask him to stand and bend his body forward over the examination table. If the patient is unable to stand, place him in a left lateral Sims' position with the knees drawn up and the buttocks near the edge of the bed or examination table.

(8) Put on a glove and spread the patient's buttocks to expose the anus and surrounding area. Asks the patient to strain as though defecating. Inspect for inflammation, discharge, lesions, scars, rectal prolapse, skin tags, and external hemorrhoids. Apply lubricant to your index finger. Explain to the patient that you will insert your gloved, lubricated finger a short distance into the rectum. Have the patient breathe through the mouth and relax.

(9) Once you have inserted your finger, rotate it to palpate all aspects of the rectal wall for nodules, tenderness, and fecal impaction. The rectal wall should feel smooth and soft. In a male patient, assess the prostate gland when palpating the anterior rectal wall; the prostate should feel firm and smooth.

h. **Genitourinary Assessment.** The male genitalia may be examined with the patient either standing or supine. However, the patient should stand as you check for hernias or varicoceles. Examine the female genitalia with the patient in a dorsal recumbent position.

(1) When assessing the urinary system, check for and evaluate edema. Press firmly over a bony surface for 5 to 10 seconds, and then remove you finger. Note how long the depression remains. Document your observation on a scale from +1 (barely detectable) to +4 (a persistent pit as deep as 1 inch). When associated with fluid retention and electrolyte imbalance, edema may indicate renal dysfunction, such as nephritis.

(2) Palpate the bladder for distention and tenderness. Press deeply in the midline about 1 to 2 inches above the symphysis pubis. During deep palpation, the patient may feel the need to urinate; this is a normal response. Note the size and location of the bladder. Check for lumps and masses. The bladder normally feels firm and relatively smooth.

(3) Ask the patient about urinary patterns such as retention, urgency and frequency. Ask the patient if he has noticed blood in his urine or if he has pain when urinating. Ask the patient to urinate into a specimen cup. Assess the sample for color, odor, and clarity.

(4) Provide the patient with a gown. and drape appropriately. ***Be sure to wear gloves.*** Expose the genitalia and inguinal areas and proceed with the examination.

(5) Inspect the inguinal and femoral areas carefully for bulges. A bulge that appears on straining suggests a hernia.

(6) Look for nits or lice at the bases of the pubic hairs.

(7) Have the male patient assume a supine position. Begin assessment of the male genital system by inspecting the penis. Look for ulcers, scars, nodules, or signs of inflammation. Compress the glans gently between your index finger and thumb to open the urethral meatus and inspect it for discharge.

(8) Inspect the scrotum. Note any swelling, lumps, or veins. Palpate each testis and epididymis. Note their size, shape, consistency, and tenderness.

(9) During the examination, the male patient may have an erection and probably be embarrassed about it. Explain to him that this is a normal response, and finish your examination in an unruffled manner.

(10) Ask the female patient to empty her bladder before you begin the examination. To assess the perineal area, position her in a dorsal recumbent position with her head and shoulders slightly elevated to relax the abdominal muscles and so that both you and the patient can see each other's face. Explain in advance what you are about to do.

(11) Assess the perineal area for character of skin and abnormal masses or discharge. Spread her labia with a gloved hand and inspect the urethral meatus; it should appear pink and free of swelling or discharge. In any patient, inflammation and discharge may signal urethral infection. Ulceration usually indicates a sexually transmitted disease.

i. **Musculoskeletal Assessment.** Musculoskeletal assessment begins the instant you see the patient. Good observation skills will enable you to gain information about muscle strength, obvious physical or functional deformities or abnormalities, and movement symmetry. If the patient's chief complaint involves a different body system, the musculoskeletal assessment should represent only a small part of the overall assessment. If the health history or physical findings suggest musculoskeletal involvement, analyze the patient's complaints and perform a complete musculoskeletal assessment.

(1) Observe the patient's general appearance, body symmetry, gait, posture, and coordination. Inspect and palpate his muscles, joints, and bones. Evaluate muscle and joint function of each body area as you proceed with the examination. Compare both sides of the body for size, strength, movement, and complaints of pain.

(2) Position the patient to allow full range of motion (ROM), but avoid tiring the patient by allowing him to sit whenever possible.

(3) Inspect spinal curvature. Have the patient stand as straight as possible and inspect the spine for alignment and the shoulders, iliac crests, and scapulae for symmetry of position and height. Normally, the thoracic spine is characterized by convex curvature and the lumbar spine is characterized by concave curvature in a standing patient. Have the patient bend forward from the waist with arms relaxed and dangling. Stand behind him and inspect the straightness of the spine, noting flank and thorax position and symmetry.

(4) Have the patient stand with his feet together. Note the relation of one knee to the other. The knees should be symmetrical and located at the same height in a forward-facing position.

(5) Ask the patient to walk away, turn around, and walk back. If the patient is elderly or infirmed, remain close and ready to help if he should stumble or start to fall. Observe and evaluate his posture, pace and length of stride, foot position, coordination, and balance. Normal findings include smooth, coordinated movements, erect posture, and 2 to 4 inches between the feet. Abnormal findings include a wide support base, arms held out to the side or in front, jerky or shuffling motions, toeing in or out, and the ball of the foot, rather than the heel, striking the floor first.

(6) To assess gross motor skills, have the patient perform range-of-motion (ROM) exercises (see Nursing Fundamentals I, figure 5-1). To assess fine motor coordination, have the patient pick up a small object from a flat surface.

(7) Assess muscle tone. Muscle tone is the tension in the resting muscle. Palpate the muscle at rest and during passive ROM from the muscle attachment at the bone to the edge of the muscle. A relaxed muscle should feel soft and pliable. A contracted muscle should feel firm.

(8) Assess muscle mass. Muscle mass is the actual size of a muscle. Assessment involves measuring the circumference of the thigh, the calf, and the upper arm. Measure at the same location on each area. Abnormal findings include circumferential differences of more than ½ inch between opposite thighs, calves and upper arms, decreased muscle size (atrophy), excessive muscle size (hypertrophy) without a history of muscle building exercises, flaccidity (atony), weakness (hypotonicity), spasticity (hypertonicity), and involuntary twitching of muscle fibers (fasciculations).

(9) Assess muscle strength and joint ROM. Have the patient perform active ROM as you apply resistance. Normally, the patient can move joints a certain distance (measured in degrees) and can easily resist pressure applied against movement. Strength is normally symmetrical. If the patient cannot perform active ROM, put the joints through passive ROM. Use a goniometer (figure 6-9) to measure the angle achieved. Place the center or zero point on the patient's joint. Place the fixed arm perpendicular to the plane of motion. As the patient moves the joint, the movable arm indicates the angle in degrees.

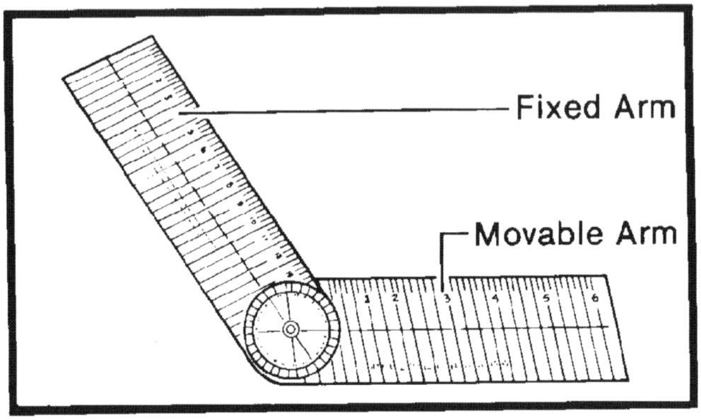


Figure 6-9. Goniometer.

j. **Assessment of the Integument.** Physical assessment of the skin, hair, and nails requires inspection and palpation. Be sure the room is warm to prevent cold-induced vasoconstriction, which may affect skin color.

(1) Systematically, assess the entire skin surface as you expose each area for inspection and palpation of other systems. Observe the patient from a distance, noting complexion, general color, and overall appearance. A bluish discoloration is due to lack of oxygen in the blood. A yellow skin tone (jaundice) indicates liver dysfunction. Note pigmentation (light and dark areas compared to the rest of the skin), freckles, and moles.

(2) Assess skin texture, consistency, temperature, moisture, and turgor. Skin texture refers to smoothness or coarseness. Consistency refers to changes in skin thickness or firmness and relates more to changes associated with lesions. The skin should feel warm to cool, and areas should feel the same bilaterally. Assess turgor by gently grasping and pulling up a fold of skin, releasing it, and observing how quickly it returns to normal shape. Normal skin usually resumes its flat shape immediately. Poor turgor may indicate dehydration and connective tissue disorders.

(3) Note the quantity, texture, color, and distribution of hair. Rub a few strands of the patient's hair between you index finger and thumb. Feel for dryness, brittleness, oiliness, and thickness.

(4) Assessment of the nails provides information about the patient's life-style, self-esteem, and level of self-care as well as health status. Inspect the nails for cleanliness, length, color, consistency, smoothness, symmetry, and for jagged or bitten edges.

(5) Note any alterations in skin integrity such as scars, rashes, sores, lesions, bruises, and discoloration. If the patient has a dressing, note the type, location, any drainage, and the amount and character of the drainage.

## 6-8. GUIDELINES FOR DOCUMENTATION

a. The nursing history and assessment should be completed for each patient within 24 hours of admission. Documentation of the physical assessment should be done in an organized fashion according to systems. Information should be thorough and flow logically from one consideration to the next. Follow general charting rules using correct medical terminology, spelling, grammar, punctuation, and authorized abbreviations. Use the proper format and write neat and legibly. Depending on ward policy, the initial physical assessment is recorded on DA Form 3888, Medical Record - Nursing History and Assessment (see figure 6-10), DA Form 3888-1, and/or SF 510, Medical Record--Nursing Notes (see figure 6-11).

b. DA Form 3888 (see figure 6-10) documents a baseline nursing history and assessment on each patient. If completed at the time of admission, it may serve as the admission-nursing note. If DA Form 3888 is completed at admission, an admission note is not needed on SF 510. Make an entry on SF 510 to refer to the DA Form 3888 for the admission note. Data entered on this form represents baseline health status information used by the nurse to plan care. (See DA Form 3888 on the following pages.)

c. The nursing assessment is reviewed and revised as additional data are collected and patient needs change. Updated nursing assessment should be documented on the SF 510. Several methods and personnel may collect patient date from which a plan of care is developed. Regardless of what data is collected, and by whom, the professional nurse is ultimately responsible for the validity and reliability of the collected data.

## 6-9. CLOSING

As you learn the techniques of performing a comprehensive patient assessment, list these techniques in the order in which they are performed. Organize the assessment in a way that limits the number of times the patient must change positions, and the number of times you must change your own position. Once you have developed an organized and systematic approach and performed the assessment a number of times, you will be able to gather both subjective and objective information quickly and effectively. This approach will provide you with the information you need to develop your nursing diagnoses and care plans.

**MEDICAL/SURGICAL ASSESSMENT**
For use of this form, see DNAP B-1

QA Appr 9 Sep 92

**MEDICAL RECORD - NURSING HISTORY AND ASSESSMENT**
For use of this form, see AR 40-407; the proponent agency is the OTSG

| 1. Date and Time of Admission | 2. Admission Diagnosis |
|---|---|
| | |

| | Yes | No | Patient's own words when possible. |
|---|---|---|---|
| 3. Tell me what you know about your illness/injury/hospitalization. | | | |
| 4. Do you have any other health problems? | | | |
| 5. Have you been hospitalized before? if so, when and for what? | | | |
| 6. What medications have you been taking? (to include prescription and over-the-counter drugs) For how long? | | | |
| 7. Are you allergic to anything? If so what? What reaction? | | | |
| 8. Do you have any special needs that require assistance with daily activities? (e.g., diet, eating, bathing, elimination, ambulating, sleeping.) Prosthetics: dentures, reading glasses, contacts. | | | |
| 9. What other concerns do you have? | | | |
| 10. How can we be most helpful? | | | |

| 11. Name of Local Contact/NOK. | 12. Relationship | 13. Telephone Number. |
|---|---|---|
| | | |

| 14. Interviewer's Signature, Rank & Title. | 15. Informant/Relationship. |
|---|---|
| | |

16. Patient Identification.

17. Personal Articles and Valuables. *(Indicate disposition of each item by initials.)*

| Item: | Bedside | Home | Treasurer | Other *(specify)* |
|---|---|---|---|---|
| | | | | |
| | | | | |
| | | | | |
| | | | | |
| | | | | |
| | | | | |
| | | | | |
| | | | | |

**DA FORM 3888, JUN 91** Replaces DA FORM 3888, AUG 79 AND DA FORM 3888-2 (TEST), AUG 85 WHICH IS OBSOLETE

**BAMC OP 505, NOV 92**

PROPONENT: DEPT OF NURS REQUIREMENT OF PRIVACY ACT OF 974 IS COVERED BY DD FORM 2005 PREVIOUS EDITIONS ARE OBSOLETE

Figure 6-10. Medical Record - Nursing History and Assessment.

**MEDICAL RECORD - NURSING HISTORY AND ASSESSMENT**

18. Additional Assessment Data.

Admission: TPR BP WT HT

ADMITTED VIA: ☐ Ambulatory ☐ Wheelchair ☐ Litter ACCOMPANIED BY: ____________

GENERAL APPEARANCE: ____________

SIGNIFICANT WEIGHT CHANGE IN PAST 3 MONTHS? ____________

MENTAL STATUS: ____________

COPING BEHAVIORS: ____________

ENVIRONMENTAL NEEDS: ☐ None ☐ Direct Observation

☐ Up Front Bed ☐ Isolation ☐ Laminar Flow

AT RISK FOR FALLS: ☐ Yes ☐ No

Refer to BAMC OP 693 on DA 4677

AT RISK FOR SKIN BREAKDOWN: ☐ Yes ☐ No

Refer to BAMC OP 634 (*PCP #13*)

PATIENT/SIGNIFICANT OTHER ORIENTED TO WARD: ☐ Yes ☐ No

PATIENT/SIGNIFICANT OTHER REVIEWED WARD RULES: ☐ Yes ☐ No

REVIEW OF SYSTEM (*as appropriate for planning care*):

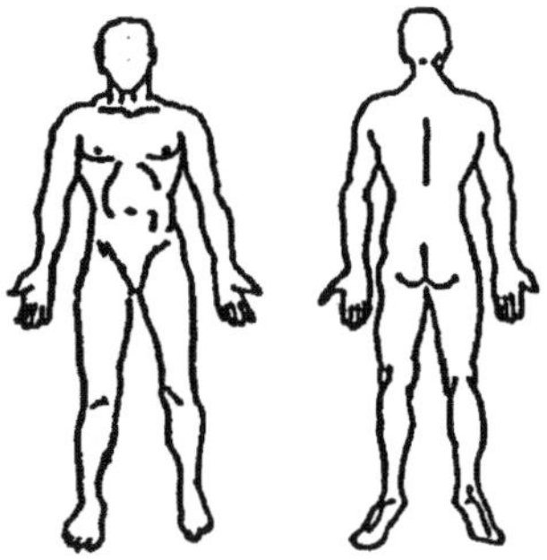

19. Typed or Printed Name of RN | 20. Signature of RN and Date/Time

ASSESSMENT CATEGORIES

1 Growth and Development

2 Neurological
- a) Orientation
- b) Level of Conciousness. alert, drowsy, lethargic, comatose, responses to verbal and painful stimuli, ability to follow commands, reflexes
- c) Describe abnormalities

3 Eyes, Ears, Nose, and Throat
- a) Eyes. Pupils, vision
- b) Ears. Hearing, drainage
- c) Rhinorrhea, nasal surgery/trauma
- d) Throat. Sore, difficulty swallowing, appearance on inspection, lymph nodes
- e) Describe abnormalities

4 Cardiovascular
- a) Skin. Color, temp, turgor, moisture
- b) Peripheral Circulation. Pulses, edema, extremities
- c) IVs. Contents of bottle hanging, bottle number, condition of site
- d) Pain. Location, radiation, duration.
- e) Intrathoracic tubes and/or dressing

5 Pulmonary
- a) Respirations. Rate, regularity, effec tiveness, depth, use of accessory muscles, nocturnal/external dyspnea. Chest movement associated with respirations.
- b) Breath sounds: Clear to auscultation Rales, Rhonchi, Wheezes, etc
- c) Oxygen. Percent given. liter/min. method of administration continuous or PRN
- d) Cough, sputum, suctioning

6 Gastrointestinal
- a) Abdominal. Auscultation (bowel sounds present), palpitation, abdominal girth measurement (if applicable)
- b) Dressings and/or drains

7 Genitourinary
- a) Urination. Continence, pattern change
- b) Female. Vaginal Discharge, LMP, last PAP smear (if applicable) etc.
- c) Male. Abnormal discharge, swelling, pain

8 Integumentary
- a) Lesions. pressure points, contractures.
- b) Color, moisture, edema, turgor, change in pigmentation

9 Musculoskeletal
- a) Movement. Purposeful/Non-purposeful. ROM. muscle strength, level of usual activity
- b) Foot care (as applicable), TED hose

10 Psycho-Social
- a) Adjustment to hospitalization and illness, manner, mood, behavior, relation to persons around them

REFERENCE: DA Pam 40-5
AMEDD Stds of Nursing Practice

REVERSE OF DA FORM 3888, JUN 91

*U.S. Government Printing Office 1991 - 281-485/40290

Figure 6-10. Medical Record - Nursing Assessment (concluded).

510-112 NSN 7540-00-634-4123

| MEDICAL RECORD | | | NURSING NOTES (Sign all notes) |
|---|---|---|---|
| DATE | HOUR | | OBSERVATIONS Include medication and treatment when indicated |
| | A.M. | P.M. | |
| | | | |
| | | | |
| | | | |
| | | | |
| | | | |
| | | | |
| | | | |
| | | | |
| | | | |
| | | | |
| | | | |
| | | | |
| | | | |
| | | | |
| | | | |
| | | | |
| | | | |
| | | | |
| | | | |
| | | | |
| | | | |
| | | | |
| | | | |
| | | | |

(Continue on reverse side)

| PATIENT'S IDENTIFICATION *(For typed or written entries give: Name—last, first, middle; grade; rank; rate; hospital or medical facility)* | REGISTER NO. | WARD NO. |
|---|---|---|

NURSING NOTES

Medical Record

STANDARD FORM 510 (REV. 7-91)
Prescribed by GSA/ICMR, FIRMR (41 CFR) 201-9.202-1

Figure 6-11. SF 510, Nursing Notes.

***Continue with Exercises***

**EXERCISE, LESSON 6**

**INSTRUCTIONS:** To complete this exercise, circle the letter of the response that best answers the question or completes the statement or write the answer in the space provided. After you have completed the all of the exercises, turn to "Solutions to Exercises" at the end of this lesson and check your answers. If you have responded to any of the exercises incorrectly, reread the material referenced after the answer.

1. Physical assessment is

   ______________________________________________

   ______________________________________________

   ______________________________________________.

2. The physical assessment is the ______________ step in the nursing process.

3. The physical assessment provides the foundation for the __________________ in which your observations play an integral part in the assessment, intervention, and evaluation phases.

4. Two purposes for a physical assessment are:

   a. ______________________________________________.

   b. ______________________________________________.

5. When preparing a patient for a physical assessment, six nursing considerations are:

   a. ______________________________________________.

   b. ______________________________________________.

   c. ______________________________________________.

   d. ______________________________________________.

   e. ______________________________________________.

   f. ______________________________________________.

6. The four basic techniques used in performing a physical assessment are:

   a. ______________________________.

   b. ______________________________.

   c. ______________________________.

   d. ______________________________.

7. Four specific areas of a general appearance and behavior assessment are:

   a. ______________________________.

   b. ______________________________.

   c. ______________________________.

   d. ______________________________.

8. One of the components of a systemic or head-to-toe physical assessment is the health history, which should clearly identify

   a. ______________________________.

   b. ______________________________.

   c. ______________________________.

**SPECIAL INSTRUCTIONS FOR EXERCISES 9 THROUGH 12.** Match the term in Column I with its definition in Column II.

| Column I | Column II |
|---|---|
| 9. ___ Vertigo | a. Ringing in the ears |
| 10. ___ Epistaxis | b. Dizziness |
| 11. ___ Accommodation | c. Nose bleeds |
| 12. ___ Tinnitus | d. Ability of the eye lens to adjust to objects at varying distances |

13. Several heart sounds can be heard by auscultation. S1, the first heart sound, is heard as ______________________________________________.

14. The second heart sound, S2, is ____________ and has a ____________________ than S1.

15. ________________________________________ should be performed before percussion and palpation because intestinal activity and bowel sounds may be altered by the motion of percussion and palpation.

16. To assess fine motor coordination, you should have the patient pick up __________ _________________________________________________________________.

17. Documentation of the physical assessment should be done in an _______________________ fashion according to ________________________.

18. The nursing history and assessment should be completed within _______ hours of admission.

***Check Your Answers on Next Page***

**SOLUTIONS TO EXERCISE, LESSON 6**

1. An organized systematic process of collecting objective data based upon a health history and head-to-toe or general systems examination. (para 6-2a)

2. first (para 6-2b)

3. Nursing care plan (para 6-2b)

4. Any two of the following are correct:
   To obtain baseline physical and mental data on the patient.
   To supplement, confirm, or question data obtained in the nursing history.
   To obtain data that will help the nurse establish nursing diagnoses and plan patient care.
   To evaluate the appropriateness of the nursing interventions in resolving the patient's identified pathophysiology problems. (paras 6-3b(1)--(4))

5. Establish a positive nurse/patient rapport.
   Explain the purpose for the physical assessment.
   Obtain an informed, verbal consent for the assessment.
   Ensure confidentiality of all data.
   Provide privacy from unnecessary exposure.
   Communicate special instructions to the patient. (paras 6-4a--f)

6. Inspection, palpation, auscultation, percussion. (paras 6-5a--d)

7. Any four of the following are correct.
   Demographic data
   Body build
   Posture and gait
   Hygiene and grooming
   Dress
   Body and breath odors
   Attitude
   Affect/mood
   Speech (paras 6-6a--h

8. The following is correct:
   - The patient's strengths and weaknesses.
   - Health risks such as hereditary and environmental factors.
   - Potential and existing health problems. (para 6-7a)

9. b (para 6-7c(3))

10 c (para 6-7c(4))

11. d (para 6-7d(2))

12 e (para 6-7c(3))

13. One dull, low-pitched sound. (para 6-7f(3))

14. Shorter; higher pitch. (para 6-7f(3))

15. Abdominal auscultation. (para 6-7g(2))

16. A small object from a flat surface. (para 6-7i(6))

17. Organized; systems. (para 6-8a)

18. 24. (para 6-8a)

***End of Lesson 6***

## LESSON ASSIGNMENT

**LESSON 7** — The Role of the Practical Nurse

TEXT ASSIGNMENT — Paragraphs 7-1 through 7-13

**LESSON OBJECTIVES** — After completing this lesson, you should be able to:

7-1. Select from a list of facts, those facts, which define, team nursing.

7-2. Identify factors related to team productivity.

7-3. Select from a list of facts, those facts that describe a manager and leader.

7-4. Select from a list of personal qualities, those that are qualities of a leader.

7-5. Identify the responsibilities of a team leader.

7-6. Identify five general facts related to patient teaching.

7-7. Identify five steps used in the teaching-learning process.

7-8. Identify factors, which affect patient learning.

7-9. Select from a list of principles, those principles of effective teaching and learning.

7-10. Identify the three types of learning.

7-11. Select from a list, the major type(s) of learning related to a specific teaching strategy.

7-12. Select from a list of guidelines, those guidelines that can help the nurse in ordering the learning experience.

**SUGGESTION** — After studying the assignment, complete the exercises at the end of this lesson. These exercises will help you to achieve the lesson objectives.

# LESSON 7

# THE ROLE OF THE PRACTICAL NURSE

## 7-1. INTRODUCTION

a. The practical nurses' role has expanded to team leadership and patient teaching. Leadership is defined as influencing individuals or groups to take an active part in the process of achieving agreed-upon goals. Nursing leadership may be defined as a process of interpersonal influence through which a patient is assisted in the establishment and achievement of goals toward improved well-being.

b. Teaching refers to activities by which specific objectives or desired behavior changes are achieved. It is an interactive process between the teacher and one or more learners. Patient teaching is inherent to the role of nursing by virtue of the nurse's position at the bedside. Shorter hospital stays which require patients to manage convalescence at home, and emphasis on health promotion and health maintenance rather than on treatment alone, have increased the need for health teaching by nurses.

## Section I. TEAM LEADERSHIP

## 7-2. TEAM NURSING

a. In 1953, Eleanor Lambertson and her colleagues proposed a system of team nursing to overcome the fragmentation of care resulting from the task-oriented functional approach. Team nursing responds to the needs of both the patient and the staff. Team members are stimulated by the team leader to learn and develop new skills. The team leader instructs the team members, supervises them, and provides assignments that offer them potential for growth. The following facts define team nursing:

(1) It is direct patient care accomplished by a specific group of nurses and allied health care workers.

(2) It is accomplished by using the nursing process.

(3) It allows for comprehensive, holistic nursing care when the team functions at a high level of efficiency.

(4) It is composed of a team leader who coordinates patient care and supervises team members, and team members who are responsible for total care given to an assigned group or number of patients.

(5) It requires cooperation and effective communication with all staff members.

b. Basic to team nursing are the team conference, nursing care plan, and leadership skills.

(1) The conference is led by the team leader, and all personnel assigned to the team should be included. The team leader should discuss the needs of the patients, establish goals, individualize the plan of care for each patient, instruct the team members, and follow up on all directions previously given to the team.

(2) The nursing care plan is a written guide that organizes information about a patient's health. It focuses on the actions that must be taken to address the patient's identified nursing diagnoses and meet the stated goals. It provides for continuity of care by a constantly changing nursing staff. The team leader starts the care plan as soon as the patient is admitted to the medical treatment facility. In response to changes in the patient's condition, and evaluation of goal achievement, the nursing care plan is updated and revised throughout the patient's hospital stay.

(3) Three leadership styles have been described: autocratic, democratic, and laissez-faire. The three are sometimes blended to fit the situation, the needs of the team leader, and/or the needs of the nursing team.

(a) Autocratic leadership. The leader determines policies and gives orders and directions to the members. Autocratic leadership often makes team members dissatisfied. It may be a necessary style when urgent decision-making is required.

(b) Democratic leadership. The leader encourages team discussion and decision-making. This supportive style increases team productivity and satisfaction. Democratic leadership has positive connotations but requires time for discussion. It may not always be the most effective method when team members lack the skills to make decisions or when urgent decision-making is required.

(c) Laissez-faire leadership. The leader participates minimally and acts as a resource person and consultant at the request of the team members. Laissez-faire leadership is described as a "hands-off" approach. It is most effective after the team has made a decision, is committed to that decision, and has the expertise to implement it.

## 7-3. FACTORS AFFECTING TEAM PRODUCTIVITY

a. Productivity implies effectiveness and efficiency in individual and group performance. To be effective, the objectives must be achieved. To be efficient, the objectives must be achieved with the least amount of resources. Productivity implies measurement. Productivity involves the relative use of skills and the relative use of knowledge. Measurement of skills work is easy, but it becomes more difficult to measure knowledge work. The 91B10 may take and record vital signs of 20 patients in one hour. The team leader may use eight hours completing next month's schedule, while directing subordinates. One difficulty in measuring the productivity of knowledge work is that often the output contributes indirectly to achieve end results. Factors affecting the nursing team's productivity are:

(1) The number of team members. A team that is too large wastes time and fosters indecision. The team should be large enough to complete the assigned tasks, but small enough for adequate communication among its members.

(2) The number of assignments. Whatever the situation, the team members must learn to organize their work so that they are able to give adequate care to all of their patients.

(3) The types of tasks to be accomplished. Team members should be competent in performing all tasks that may be assigned. Non-nursing tasks such as answering the telephone, emptying the garbage, and transporting non-acute patients should be eliminated from their duties.

(4) The time allocated to complete the tasks. As conservation of scarce resources such as time, money, and supplies is more vigorously enforced, the need for nurses to be "faster and smarter" in delivering patient care will increase.

(5) The environment. A smaller staff will be on duty during the evening and night. There will be fewer members to a team, and each member will be assigned to care for more patients. Although more personnel are available during the day shift, more patient services are provided. Continuity of care is the key; communication between shifts is vital.

(6) The management style of the team leader. Whether the team leader has an autocratic, democratic, or laissez-faire management style, he must have a thorough knowledge of nursing and an intuitive understanding of human behavior if the team is to produce efficiently.

(7) The skills and experience of each team member. Each team member should have the needed skills for the technique, treatment, or procedure they are to perform. If in doubt, they should know where to find the SOP (standing operating procedures) if required.

b. Although the terms management and leadership are sometimes treated as synonyms, there is a distinct difference between a manager and a leader. The key functions of a manager are planning, organizing, staffing, leading, and controlling. Leadership is an important aspect of managing; however, there can be leaders of completely unorganized groups.

(1) A manager plans and sets up the organizational structure and assigns specific people to accomplish specific tasks.

(2) A leader influences people to be enthusiastic and willing to achieve the desired goals. Leadership and motivation are closely connected.

(3) Team leadership requires some management skills as well as leadership skills.

## 7-4. LEADERSHIP QUALITIES

a. Although many great nursing leaders emerged in the past, most nurses were kept in subordinate positions. This subordination has diminished as more nurses learn to apply their leadership skills to attain the ultimate goal of improved patient care. Nurses with leadership skills can effect desired changes in the patient's health patterns, in the medical treatment facility, in the nursing profession, and in the community.

b. Many adjectives are used to describe the traits or qualities of a leader. With education, training, and practice, every nurse can develop the following leadership qualities.

(1) Professional knowledge. Nursing involves knowledge in biology, nursing science, social science, and many other areas. It is impossible to master them all. Learn how to find and use appropriate reference materials and resource persons quickly and efficiently. Keep up with current nursing practices for validity, reliability, and applicability and share your knowledge with peers and subordinates. Political awareness is also required. Know how local, state, and national level legislation will affect health care before supporting candidates or voting. Good leaders must be advocates of patient's rights in order to improve patient care.

(2) A positive self-image. Leaders must be enthusiastic, dynamic, and self-directed. They must be comfortable with themselves and act as role models to followers.

(3) Effective communication. Leaders must communicate effectively in order to relate to others. The ability to communicate effectively is especially needed when relating to patients, peers, subordinates, and superiors. Effective communication skills are used to:

(a) Share information with team members and involve them in the decision-making process.

(b) Define specific expectations.

(c) Offer suggestions and assistance in the completion of tasks.

(d) Elicit feedback from team members and provide feedback to superiors.

(e) Give constructive criticism and offer positive reinforcement to subordinates.

(f) Practice active listening.

(4) Assertiveness. Leaders need to be assertive in team interaction and other leadership situations. Assertiveness is used extensively when effecting change. Many nurses participate in assertiveness training programs so they can strengthen the position of nursing in the health-care system and increase its influence on patient care.

(5) Flexibility. Changes in the needs of patients, families, and the nursing team can occur within minutes. The nursing role and all nursing functions require flexibility.

(6) An understanding of human needs. The highest level on Maslow's hierarchy of needs is self-actualization, which is the need for an individual to reach his or her potential through full development of their unique capabilities. Effective leaders seek ways to promote self-actualization in themselves and team members. An effective leader understands the human need to feel useful and important, and the desire to belong, and to be recognized as an individual.

## 7-5. TEAM LEADER RESPONSIBILITIES

a. The National Federation of Licensed Practical Nurses (NFLPN) Revised Statement of Functions and Qualifications of the Licensed Practical Nurse states that the licensed practical nurse, with additional preparation in specialized areas and under direction of autonomous health professionals, is qualified to:

(1) Supervise other nursing and health-related personnel.

(2) Coordinate and make assignments of other nursing and health-related personnel and patients.

(3) Serve as team leader.

(4) Serve as charge nurse.

b. All members on a nursing team work together under the direction of the physician to help the patient return to his optimum function as quickly as possible. The team leader's responsibilities are:

(1) To attend change of shift reports. The change of shift report may be given to the entire oncoming shift in one area or it may be given in "walking rounds." In walking rounds, the departing nurse moves from patient to patient as he or she gives the report to the oncoming staff. This enables the oncoming staff to view the patient's equipment and dressings as the departing nurse reports what has occurred during her shift.

(2) To assign personnel. Personnel assignments are made with the patient's needs and each team member's proficiency in mind. The team leader reviews the nursing care plan, provides each team member with a written assignment sheet, and discusses the assignment with each member. The team leader also assigns breaks and lunch time.

(3) To assist team members with patient care. The team leader may assist with patient care as needed, but usually supervises the care that team members provide and sees that the goals of patient care are being met. He explains procedures to team members.

(4) To coordinate staff activities. The team leader coordinates staff activities to ensure quality patient care. The team leader attends patient care conferences and provides input to the Nursing Care Plan. He keeps abreast of any changes in patient status. He ensures utilization of quality assurance and infection control policies.

(5) To motivate the team. The team leader motivates the team to give skilled nursing care. Self-esteem, status, affiliation with others, affection, giving, accomplishment, and self-assertion are regarded as secondary needs. These needs vary in intensity with various individuals. The team leader must do or say those things, which will influence the team members to act in the desired manner (give skilled nursing care).

(6) To make final rounds. About one hour before the shift ends, the team leader should begin final rounds to observe and assess patient care and patient needs, and to see that everything is in order before the staff goes off duty for that shift. In making final rounds, the team leader would include the following:

(a) Check for completion of assignments.

(b) Check input/output (I&O) sheets.

(c) Check intravenous (IV) infusions and nasogastric (NG) intubations.

(d) Review nursing documentation.

(e) Talk to the patients. Gather information for the change of shift report. Listen for compliments or complaints concerning nursing care.

(f) Thank team members and give constructive feedback to those team members who were unable to complete their assignments.

(7) To complete nursing care rounds. The team leader should visually assess individual patients following the change of shift report.

## Section II. PATIENT TEACHING

### 7-6. FACTS RELATED TO PATIENT TEACHING

a. Patient teaching is a function of nursing and a legal requirement of nursing personnel. Teaching is considered a function of nursing. In some states teaching is included in the legal definition of nursing, making it a required function of nursing personnel by law.

b. Patient teaching is defined as a system of activities intended to produce learning. These activities should help the patient meet individual learning objectives. If they do not, the patient's need should be reassessed and the activities replaced by others. For example, explanation alone may not teach a diabetic patient how to prepare the syringe for an injection. Actually preparing the syringe may be more effective.

c. Patient teaching is a dynamic interaction between the nurse (teacher) and the patient (learner). Both the teacher and the learner communicate information, emotions, perceptions, and attitudes to the other.

d. Before learning can occur, a relationship of trust and respect must exist between the teacher and learner. The learner trusts the teacher to have the required knowledge and skills to teach and the teacher respects the learner's ability to reach the goals. This relationship is enhanced by communication that is continuous and reciprocal, once mutual trust and respect have been established.

e. The goal of patient teaching is the patient's active participation in health care and his compliance with instructions. Once the nurse begins instructing a patient (or family/support persons), the teaching process should continue until the participants reach the goals, change the goals, or decide that the goals will not help meet the learning objectives.

### 7-7. STEPS IN THE TEACHING-LEARNING PROCESS

a. Assess the Patient's Learning Needs.

(1) Use all appropriate sources of information. Review the patient's medical records. Read the history of medical problems as well as diagnoses, physical examinations, documentation of the nursing assessment, and the nursing interventions that have been performed. The patient and the family or support persons are the best source of needs assessment information.

(2) Identify the knowledge, attitude, or skills needed by the patient or family/support persons. Learning can be divided into three domains: cognitive, affective, and psychomotor. You may categorize learning that is planned for the patient into these three areas.

(a) Cognitive involves the storing and recalling of new knowledge and information.

(b) Affective learning includes changes in attitudes, values, and feelings.

(c) Psychomotor learning has occurred when a physical skill has been acquired.

(3) Assess emotional and experiential readiness to learn. Readiness is not the patient's physical ability to learn. The readiness to learn in an adult may be related to a social role. Being assured that they are partners in the teaching-learning process gives adult learners the sense of control that they are accustomed to in their daily living.

(4) Assess the patient's ability to learn. The teaching approach must be appropriate to the developmental stage of the learner. You should assess the patient's intellectual development, motor development, psychosocial development, and emotional maturity. Chronological age does not guarantee maturity.

(5) Identify the patient's strengths. Learning strengths are the patient's personal resources such as psychomotor skills, above-average comprehension, reasoning, memory, or successful learning in the past. For example, if the patient knows how to cook, this knowledge can be useful when learning about a special diet.

(6) Use anticipatory guidance. Anticipatory guidance focuses on psychologically preparing a person for an unfamiliar or painful event. When patients know what to expect, anxiety is reduced and they are able to cope more effectively.

b. Diagnose the Learning Needs. Be realistic. When a lack of knowledge, attitude, or skill hinders a patient's self-promotion of health, the nurse diagnoses the deficit. Confirm your diagnosis with the family. In addition, assess your own knowledge base and teaching skills. You teach information and skills to patients which you lack.

c. Develop a Teaching Plan. Planning ensures the most efficient use of your time and increases the patient's chances for learning. A teaching plan follows the steps of the nursing process.

(1) Develop measurable learner objectives for each diagnosis of a learning need.

(a) Identify short-term and long-term objectives.

(b) Prioritize the objectives.

(c) Determine who should be included in the teacher-learning process (family members, friends, or other support persons). For example, the person who cooks for the patient is asked to participate in any nutritional teaching.

(d) Include the patient in planning. Ask his permission to involve family members or others.

(2) Create a teaching plan. One nurse or several nurses can prepare and use a teaching plan. There are standardized teaching plans available for major topics of health teaching (some for computer use). Individualize the standardized plans to the patient's needs and abilities.

(a) Match content with the appropriate teaching strategies and learner activities. For example, content explaining why certain treatments and medications are needed may be matched with printed or audiovisual materials. Children respond well to teaching strategies that permit them to participate actively.

(b) Schedule teaching within the limits of time constraints. Shorter, more frequent sessions allow the patient to digest the new information and prevents him from becoming tired or uncomfortable due to his illness.

(c) Decide on group or individual teaching and formal or informal teaching. Some learner objectives are met more readily in a one-to-one encounter (i.e., colostomy care) while others are met more easily in a group discussion with other patients that have similar problems. Formal teaching is the planned teaching done to fulfill learner objectives. Informal teaching occurs during nursing interactions with the patient and his family. Informal teaching often leads to planned, formal sessions.

(d) Formulate a verbal or written contract with the patient. The contract is informal and is not legally binding; however, such an agreement serves to motivate both the patient and the nurse to attain the learning objectives. It points out the responsibilities of both the nurse (teacher) and the patient (learner). Whether verbal or written, the contract should not be intimidating, but viewed as an aid to learning. Failure to meet contracted objectives should be redirected into new learning and decision-making situations.

d. Implement the Teaching Plan. The implementation phase may be only a few minutes or the sessions may extend over a period of days, or perhaps months. Use interpersonal skills as well as effective communication techniques. Do not use technical and medical terms unless the patient has a medical background, but avoid a condescending attitude. Your attitude has a greater effect on the patient than any other factor. If the patient must learn special techniques or procedures, tell him or her that it takes time and practice to perform these new skills confidently. Review the contractual agreement before implementing the teaching plan.

**CONTRACT AGREEMENT**

I will participate in the learning activities planned to help me learn about a low cholesterol diet. While hospitalized, I will read the materials given to me and ask questions if I do not understand. I will cooperate with the dietitian, CPT Meaney, and the nurse, SFC B. Wellman, in planning my meals. If I need help when I get home, I will call SFC Wellman

Julie Davis

I will provide Julie Davis with the activities necessary for her to follow a low cholesterol diet accurately.

B. Wellman, LPN

Figure 7-1. Example of a contractual agreement.

(1) Prepare the physical environment. It should be a nonthreatening atmosphere, free of distractions and interruptions. Ensure adequate space and lighting, comfortable chairs, good ventilation, and privacy.

(2) Gather all teaching aids: posters, printed material, audiovisual material, and equipment if needed.

(3) Deliver content in an organized manner using planned teaching strategies. If you are teaching a skill or procedure, follow the correct sequence so that the patient is not confused.

(4) Be flexible. Observe the patient for clues or additional assessment data that could alter the original teaching plan. Adapt or reorganize the teaching plan if necessary.

e. Evaluate the Teaching-Learning. Do not assume that learning has occurred without feedback. The key is to write measurable learner objectives in the teaching plan that describe the desired behavior.

(1) Evaluate whether learner objectives have been met. There are several ways to do this.

(a) Observation. Observe the patient to verify that he has put the information that he learned into practice.

(b) Patient's comments. The patient will usually state whether or not he or she understands the information being taught.

(c) Direct questions. Ask the patient a question requiring a response, which reflects his or her level of knowledge about the topic.

(d) Return demonstration. Have the patient perform the procedure as it was demonstrated. This is an excellent method of evaluating proficiency in psychomotor skills.

(2) Evaluate teaching. Immediately after each session, evaluate your teaching effectiveness.

(a) Quickly review how implementation of the plan went and mentally make note of both your strengths and weaknesses.

(b) Seek feedback from the patients. Use a simple questionnaire with space for comments but one, which requires only check marks to answer. The questionnaires may be more honest and helpful if anonymous.

(3) Revise the teaching plan. Evaluation may reveal that the teaching plan should be revised. Revision is part of the teaching-learning process; it is not an indication of failure. Make adjustments accordingly to meet the patient's needs.

(a) Alter the content and teaching strategies if the objectives were unrealistic, the content too complex, or the teaching strategy inappropriate.

(b) Employ motivational counseling if the patient is unwilling to participate in learning activities or to learn how to care for himself.

(c) Reschedule teaching sessions if the time and frequency of sessions affected the teacher-learner process.

(4) Document the teaching-learning process. Teaching is an important and required nursing responsibility; it must be documented in the patient's record.

(a) Include a summary of the diagnosed learning needs, the teaching plan, implementation of the plan, and evaluation results.

(b) Show evidence in the evaluation statement that learning has occurred, or how the problem was resolved if the patient or support person did not learn the material taught.

## 7-8. FACTORS WHICH AFFECT LEARNING

a. Factors, which affect patient learning, need to be assessed in order for appropriate teaching strategies to be used.

b. Include the following factors in your assessment.

(1) Developmental considerations. Knowledge of intellectual, psychosocial, and physiologic age is necessary before you select age-appropriate teaching methods. Delayed development in any of these areas should be considered.

(a) Children have limited past experiences. Adults learn more quickly than children because they are able to build upon previous knowledge.

(b) Use chronological age to assess whether the developmental stage is as would be expected.

(2) Educational level. You will effectively promote learning if you are aware of the learner's intellectual ability and avoid "talking down" to him or her or using an inappropriate teaching strategy.

(3) Past learning experiences. Attitudes toward future learning are influenced by learning experiences in the past. Encourage the learner to express how he views education so that you can deal with his feelings before teaching is attempted.

(4) Physical condition. The patient will not be ready to learn until he is comfortable enough to pay attention to the information you present.

(5) Sensory abilities. Note any deficit in the learner's sight, hearing, and touch so that teaching is planned appropriately.

(6) Emotional health. The emotional state of the learner should be conducive to learning before teaching is done.

(a) A patient, who is moderately anxious about his/her condition, will probably be attentive to presentation of information that will help him manage the condition.

(b) If the patient is in a state of crisis with a high level of anxiety, delay teaching until the crisis is over.

(7) Social and economic stability. Being hospitalized and absent from work cause some patients excessive stress. Help the patient deal with any social and economic problems before imposing the additional stress of learning information or a new skill.

(8) Responsibility. To learn self-care or take preventive measures against illness, a patient must have a sense of responsibility. Encourage the patient to participate in planning the learning activities to promote his feelings of control.

(9) Self perception. Self-perception has an effect on the ability to learn. If effective learning about a health problem is to occur, any unrealistic self-image or body image should be addressed. If necessary, help the patient improve self-image before focusing on learning needs.

(10) Attitude toward learning. Attitude toward learning is difficult to measure. Talk to the patient to get an idea of how he feels about learning to improve his health. If the patient has a negative attitude about learning, establish a relationship that will help in altering that attitude.

(11) Motivation to learn. The patient must want to learn for teaching to be effective. If the patient is not motivated to learn the material needed to improve his health, discussing his interest and concerns may lead to success.

(12) Culture. Some cultures value education that will improve their condition, while others view change or new practices as threatening. Do not stereotype any person because of his culture; but recognize that each person has a unique family background with certain cultural values that may have an effect on how teaching learning is perceived.

(13) Communication skills. The basic requirement for the teaching-learning process is communication. Assess your communication skills as well as those of the learner.

(a) Assess the learner's reading skills before using printed material as a teaching aid.

(b) Assess to what degree English is spoken and understood by the learner. Most hospitals have printed and audiovisual materials available for non-English speaking patients.

## 7-9. PRINCIPLES FOR EFFECTIVE TEACHING-LEARNING

a. These basic principles are effective guidelines when applied in situations in which the teaching-learning process is used by nurses to meet the needs of clients.

**NOTE:** Clients may be patients, family members, or support persons.

(1) The teaching-learning process is facilitated by the existence of a helping relationship.

(a) A helping relationship exist among people who provide and receive assistance in meeting a common goal. The relationship is established as a result of communication.

(b) The communication is continuous and reciprocal.

(2) Nurses in the role of teachers must be able to communicate effectively with individuals, with small groups, and in some instances with large groups.

(3) Knowledge of the communication process is necessary for the assessment of verbal and nonverbal feedback.

(4) A thorough assessment of clients and the factors affecting learning helps to diagnose their learning needs accurately.

(5) The teaching-learning process is more effective when the client is included in the planning of learner objectives.

(6) Unless the client values these objectives, little learning is likely to occur.

(7) The implementation of a teaching plan should include varied strategies for sensory stimulation, which apparently promote learning.

(8) Relating new learning material to clients' past life experiences is effective in helping to assimilate new knowledge.

(9) Proposed behavioral changes must always be realistic and explored in the context of the client's resources and everyday life-style.

(10) Careful attention should be paid to time constraints, scheduling, and the physical environment.

(11) Learner objectives provide the basis for evaluating whether learning has occurred.

(12) When learning objectives have not been met, careful reassessment provides ideas for changing the teaching plan for subsequent implementation.

b. The teaching-learning process and the nursing process are interdependent. Patient teaching is approached more effectively if the steps of the nursing process are followed.

## 7-10. TYPES OF LEARNING

a. Three domains, or types of learning, have been identified as cognitive, affective, and psychomotor.

(1) The cognitive domain includes intellectual skills such as thinking, knowing, and understanding. When the patient stores and recalls information, he is using the cognitive domain. For example, after attending classes on the low sodium diet a patient states how salt affects the blood pressure.

(2) The affective domain includes feelings, emotions, interests, attitudes, and appreciations. An example would be a patient's acceptance of having a colostomy and maintaining his self-esteem.

(3) The psychomotor domain involves motor skills. An example would be a patient demonstrating clean technique when changing her dressing.

b. Nurses should include each of these three domains in patient teaching plans (see paragraph 7-7a(2)).

## 7-11. SELECTING TEACHING STRATEGIES

a. Consider the different teaching strategies during the planning stage and choose a method of teaching that is suited to the individual being taught, for the material to be learned, and for you, the teacher.

b. Consider the content and the types of learning. The content to be taught is determined by the objectives. For example, when teaching self-care to a recently diagnosed diabetic, one of the objectives may be "Identify appropriate sites for insulin injections." This means that you must include content about body sites suitable for insulin injections. You should have some knowledge of sources for content information as a result of your own education and training.

c. Consider the following in matching sources of content information with a suitable strategy for the individual learner and for you, the nurse-teacher:

(1) A person who cannot read needs a source of content material in other than printed form. Use of games and role-play are popular and fun ways for children to learn.

(2) Discussion is not the best strategy for teaching a psychomotor skill. Demonstration of techniques using a practice model is an effective way of teaching someone to give an injection.

(3) Some people are visually oriented and learn best through seeing. Others learn best through hearing; an explanation or one-on-one discussion may be the most suited method.

(4) The nurse-teacher must be a competent group leader to use group discussion as a teaching strategy.

d. Some methods are better suited to certain learning objectives than others. A 10-year old recovering from burns as a result of playing with matches would be receptive to a comic book on personal safety; an adult burn victim could learn similar information by discussing safety measures. Use of a variety of teaching strategies aids learning. See Table 7-1 for selected teaching strategies for the three types of learning and characteristics of each strategy.

## 7-12. SEQUENCING THE LEARNING EXPERIENCES

a. Whether formal or informal, teaching requires a plan or it becomes haphazard and the patient's need for information goes unattended. The following guidelines are helpful in sequencing or ordering the learning experiences.

(1) Learning is facilitated when there is some personal interest. Start with something the learner has identified as a need or concern. For example, before he learns how to administer insulin to himself, an adolescent is seeking information on adjusting his lifestyle so that he can still play football.

(2) Start with what the learner knows and proceed to the unknown. If you do not know the patient's knowledge or skill level, illicit this information by asking questions or having the patient complete a form.

(3) Teach an area that is anxiety provoking first, if the learner has a high level of anxiety that can impair concentration in other areas. For example, women cannot concentrate on learning to bath her husband in bed because she is highly anxious about being able to move him and turn him in bed.

| STRATEGY | TYPE OF LEARNING | CHARACTERISTICS |
|---|---|---|
| Explanation or description (for example, lecture) | Cognitive | Teacher controls content and pace.<br>Feedback is determined by teacher.<br>May be given to individual or group.<br>Encourages retention of facts. |
| One-on-one discussion | Affective, Cognitive | Encourages participation by learner.<br>Permits reinforcement and repetition at learner's level.<br>Permits introduction of sensitive subjects |
| Answering questions | Cognitive | Teacher controls most of content and pace.<br>Teacher must understand question and what it means to learner.<br>Can be used with individuals and groups.<br>Teacher sometimes needs to confirm whether question has been answered by asking learner, "Does that answer your question?" |
| Demonstration | Psychomotor | Often used with explanation.<br>Can be used with individuals, small groups, or large groups.<br>Does not permit use of equipment by learners. |
| Group discussion | Affective, Cognitive | Learner can obtain assistance from supportive group.<br>Group members learn from one another. |
| Practice | Psychomotor | Allows repetition and immediate feedback.<br>Permits "hands-on" experience. |
| Printed and audiovisual materials | Cognitive | Forms include, books, pamphlets, films, programmed instruction, and computer learning.<br>Learners can proceed at their own speed.<br>Nurse-teacher can act as resource person.<br>Need not be present during learning. |
| Role playing | Affective, Cognitive | Permits expression of attitudes, values, and emotions.<br>Can assist in development of communication skills.<br>Involves active participation by learner. |
| Modeling | Affective, Psychomotor | Nurse sets example by attitude, psychomotor skills. |

Table 7-1. Selected teaching strategies.

(4) Teach the basic concepts first when there are variations or adjustments in a procedure, then proceed to the variations or adjustments. Learners may become confused if they have to consider variations and adjustments before understanding the basic concepts of a procedure. For example, teach a patient how to insert a Foley catheter before teaching him what to do if the catheter stops draining.

**7-13. CLOSING**

The role of the practical nurse varies with the situation. Practical nurses actively participate as team leaders, managers, and teachers. The traditional skills of nurses were psychomotor skills involving use of the hands. Individualizing care and communicating activities require nurses to use affective skills. Cognitive skills are required in all aspects of the nursing process. These expanded nursing roles have established new dimensions for nursing practice.

Continue with Exercises

## EXERCISE, LESSON 7

**INSTRUCTIONS**: To complete this exercise, circle the letter of the response that best answers the question or completes the statement or write the answer in the space provided. After you have completed the all of the exercises, turn to "Solutions to Exercises" at the end of this lesson and check your answers. If you have responded to any of the exercises incorrectly, reread the material referenced after the answer.

1. Leadership is defined as ______________________________________________
______________________________________________________________________.

2. Teaching refers to activities by which ___________________________________
_________________________________________________ are achieved.

3. List five facts that define team nursing.

    a. ________________________________________________________________
    ________________________________________________________________
    ________________________________________________________________.

    b. ________________________________________________________________
    ________________________________________________________________
    ________________________________________________________________.

    c. ________________________________________________________________
    ________________________________________________________________
    ________________________________________________________________.

    d. ________________________________________________________________
    ________________________________________________________________
    ________________________________________________________________.

    e. ________________________________________________________________
    ________________________________________________________________
    ________________________________________________________________.

**SPECIAL INSTRUCTIONS FOR EXERCISES 4 THROUGH 6.** Three leadership styles have been described. Match each description of leadership styles in Column I with the appropriate leader style in Column II.

| Column I | | Column II |
|---|---|---|
| 4. _____ | The leader participates minimally and acts as a resource person and consultant at the request of the team members. | a. Autocratic |
| | | b. Democratic |
| 5. _____ | The leader determines policy and gives orders and directions to the members. | c. Laissez-faire |
| 6. _____ | The leader encourages team discussion and decision making. | |

7. List seven factors affecting the nursing team's productivity.

   a. ________________________________________.

   b. ________________________________________.

   c. ________________________________________.

   d. ________________________________________.

   e. ________________________________________.

   f. ________________________________________.

   g. ________________________________________.

8. Productivity implies ____________________ and ____________________ in individual and group performance.

9. The key functions of a manager are:

   a. _______________________________.

   b. _______________________________.

   c. _______________________________.

   d. _______________________________.

   e. _______________________________.

10. A completely unorganized group cannot have a leader.

   a. True.

   b. False.

11. A leader ______________________ people to be enthusiastic and willing to ____________________________________________________________.

12. List six personal qualities of a leader.

   a. _______________________________.

   b. _______________________________.

   c. _______________________________.

   d. _______________________________.

   e. _______________________________.

   f. _______________________________.

13. All members of a nursing team work together. The team leader's responsibilities are to:

a. ________________________________________________.

b. ________________________________________________.

c. ________________________________________________.

d. ________________________________________________.

e. ________________________________________________.

f. ________________________________________________.

g. ________________________________________________.

14. Patient teaching is a function of nursing and a ____________________ requirement of nursing personnel.

15. Before learning can occur, a relationship of ______________________________ must exist between the teacher and learner.

16. The goal of patient teaching is ________________________________________ ________________________________________________________________.

17. Once the nurse begins instructing a patient, the teaching process should continue until:

a. Participants decide that the goals will not help meet the learning objectives.

b. Participants change the goals.

c. Participants reach the goals.

d. All of the above.

18. List five steps used in the teaching-learning process.

a. ______________________________.

b. ______________________________.

c. ______________________________.

d. ______________________________.

e. ______________________________.

19. For appropriate teaching strategies to be used, factors that affect patient learning, need to be assessed. List any six of these factors.

a. ______________________________.

b. ______________________________.

c. ______________________________.

d. ______________________________.

e. ______________________________.

f. ______________________________.

20. Which of the following is <u>not</u> one of the basic principles for effective teaching learning?

a. The teaching-learning process is facilitated by the existence of a helping relationship.

b. Nurses in the role of teachers must be able to communicate effectively with individuals, with small groups, and in some instances with large groups.

c. Knowledge of the communication process is not necessary for the nurse-teacher to assess feedback.

d. The teaching-learning process is more effective when the client is included in the planning of learner objectives.

21. One principle for effective teaching-learning is that proposed behavioral changes must be ________________________ and explored in the context of the client's ________________________________________________________.

22. Three domains or types of learning have been identified as

a. ______________________________________________.

b. ______________________________________________.

c. ______________________________________________.

23. List the major type(s) of learning related to the following teaching strategies.

a. Explanation or description __________________.

b. Modeling __________________.

c. Demonstration __________________.

d. One-on-one discussion __________________.

24. When selecting teaching strategies, you should consider the content and the types of learning. The content to be taught is determined by the _________________.

25. In ordering or sequencing the learning experiences, one guideline that may be helpful is to start with something the ________________ has identified as a need or concern.

26. Another guideline in sequencing learning experiences is you should teach any area that is anxiety-provoking ____________.

27. When there are variations or adjustments in a procedure, you should teach the ________________________________ first.

Check Your Answers on Next Page

**SOLUTIONS TO EXERCISE, LESSON 7**

1. Influencing individuals or groups to take an active part in the process of achieving agreed-upon goals. (para 7-1a)

2. Specific objectives or desired behavior changes. (para 7-1b)

3. It is direct patient care accomplished by a specific group of nurses and allied health care workers.
   It is accomplished by using the nursing process.
   It allows for comprehensive, holistic nursing care when the team functions at a high level of efficiency.
   It is composed of a team leader who coordinates patient care and supervises team members, and team members who are responsible for total care given to an assigned group or number of patients.
   It requires cooperation and effective communication with all staff members. (paras 7-2a(1)--(5))

4. c (para 7-2b(3))

5. a (para 7-2b(3))

6 b (para 7-2b(3))

7. Any four of the following are correct.
   The number of team members.
   The number of assignments.
   The types of tasks to be accomplished.
   The time allocated to complete the tasks.
   The environment.
   The management style of the team leader.
   The skills and experience of each team member. (paras 7-3a(1)--(7))

8. Effectiveness; efficiency (para 7-3a)

9. The following, in any order, are correct.
   Planning.
   Organizing
   Staffing.
   Leading.
   Controlling. (para 7-3b)

10. b. (para 7-3b)

11. Influences; achieve the desired goals. (para 7-3b(2))

12. Professional knowledge.
    A positive self-image.
    Effective communication.
    Assertiveness.
    Flexibility.
    An understanding of human need. (paras 7-4b(1)--(6))

13. Attend change of shift reports.
    Assign personnel.
    Assist team members with patient care.
    Coordinate staff activities.
    Motivate the team.
    Make final rounds.
    Complete nursing care rounds. (paras 7-5b(1)--(7))

14. Legal. (para 7-6a)

15. Trust and respect. (para 7-6d)

16. The patient's active participation in health care and his compliance with instructions. (para 7-6e)

17. d. (para 7-6e)

18. Assess the patient's learning needs.
    Diagnose the learning needs.
    Develop a teaching plan.
    Implement the teaching plan.
    Evaluate the teaching-learning. (paras 7-7a--e)

19. Any six of the following are correct.
    Developmental considerations.
    Education level.
    Past learning experiences.
    Physical condition.
    Sensory abilities.
    Emotional health.
    Social and economic stability.
    Responsibility.
    Self-perception.
    Attitude toward learning.
    Motivation to learn.
    Culture.
    Communication skills. (paras 7-8b(1)--(13))

20. c (paras 7-9a(1)--(5))

21. Realistic; the client's resources and everyday lifestyle. (para 7-9a(9))

22. Cognitive
Affective
Psychomotor. (para 7-10a)

23. a. Cognitive.
    b. Affective, psychomotor.
    c. Psychomotor.
    d. Affective, cognitive. (Table 7-1)

24. Objectives. (para 7-11b)

25. Learner. (para 7-12a(2))

26. First. (para 7-12a(3))

27. Basic content. (para 7-12a(4))

End of Lesson 7

## LESSON ASSIGNMENT

**LESSON 8** Perioperative Patient Care.

**TEXT ASSIGNMENT** Paragraphs 8-1 through 8-25.

**LESSON OBJECTIVES** After completing this lesson, you should be able to:

8-1. Select from a list of facts, those facts related to the surgical experience.

8-2. Identify items found on DD Form 1924, Surgical Check List.

8-3. Identify nursing implications related to preoperative preparation of a patient.

8-4. Select from a list, the definition of perioperative patient care.

8-5. Select from descriptive statements, the key members of the surgical team.

8-6. Identify nine factors, which effect selection of an anesthetic agent.

8-7. Identify three factors the anesthesiologist/anesthetist considers when selecting an anesthetic agent.

8-8. Identify three major classifications of anesthetic agents.

8-9. Select from a list, the descriptor for the purpose of surgical intervention.

8-10. Select from a list, complications which should be prevented in the recovery room.

8-11. Select from a list of facts, those facts related to respiratory distress.

8-12. Identify nursing implications related to the prevention of respiratory distress.

8-13. Select from a list of facts, those facts related to hypovolemic shock.

8-14. Identify nursing implications related to the detection of pending hypovolemic shock.

8-15. Identify nursing implications related to the general care of a patient in the recovery room.

8-16. Select from a list, the effects of anesthesia during the postoperative period.

8-17. Select from a list, possible negative effects of surgery on the integumentary system.

8-18. Match the type of postoperative wound closure and the appropriate healing processes.

8-19. Select from a list of factors, those factors that may impair wound healing.

8-20. Given a description of wound drains, select the type of wound drain described.

8-21. Identify nursing implications related to the care of a postoperative patient according to body systems or related to the care of a postoperative patient in general.

**SUGGESTION**

After studying the assignment, complete the exercises at the end of this lesson. These exercises will help you to achieve the lesson objectives.

# LESSON 8

# PERIOPERATIVE PATIENT CARE

## 8-1. INTRODUCTION

a. Perioperative refers to the total span of surgical intervention. Surgical intervention is a common treatment for injury, disease, or disorder. The surgeon *intervenes* in the disease process by repairing, removing, or replacing body tissues or organs. Surgery is *invasive* because an incision is made into the body or a part of the body is removed.

b. Perioperative patient care is a variety of nursing activities carried out before, during, and after surgery. The perioperative period has three phases:

(1) The ***preoperative phase*** begins with the decision that surgical intervention is necessary and ends when the patient is transferred to the operating room table.

(2) The ***intraoperative phase*** is the period during which the patient is undergoing surgery in the operating room. It ends when the patient is transferred to the post-anesthesia recovery room.

(3) The ***postoperative phase*** lasts from the patient's admission to the recovery room through the complete recovery from surgery.

## 8-2. THE SURGICAL EXPERIENCE

a. Surgery is classified as ***major*** or ***minor*** based on the degree of risk for the patient. Surgery may be classified as *elective*, meaning that it is necessary but scheduled at the convenience of the patient and the health care provider. When surgery must be done immediately to save the patient's life, a body part, or bodily function, it is classified as ***emergency surgery***. Regardless of whether the surgery is major or minor, elective or emergency, it requires both physical and psychosocial adaptation for the patient and his family. It is an important event in a person's life.

(1) Minor surgery is brief, carries a low risk, and results in few complications. It may be performed in an outpatient clinic, same-day surgery setting, or in the operating suite of a hospital.

(2) Major surgery requires hospitalization, is usually prolonged, carries a higher degree of risk, involves major body organs or life-threatening situations, and has the potential of postoperative complications.

b. Surgery produces physical stress relative to the extent of the surgery and the injury to the tissue involved. Surgical intervention may be for one or more reasons. The following descriptors classify surgical procedures by purpose:

(1) Ablative--removal of a diseased organ or structure (e.g., appendectomy).

(2) Diagnostic--removal and examination of tissue (e.g., biopsy).

(3) Constructive--repair a congenitally malformed organ or tissue. (e.g., harelip; cleft palate repair).

(4) Reconstructive--repair or restoration of an organ or structure (e.g., colostomy; rhinoplasty, cosmetic improvement).

(5) Palliative--relief of pain (for example, rhizotomy--interruption of the nerve root between the ganglion and the spinal cord).

(6) Transplant--transfer an organ or tissue from one body part to another, or from one person to another, to replace a diseased structure, to restore function, or to change appearance (for example, kidney, heart transplant; skin graft).

c. The physical stress of surgery is greatly magnified by the psychological stress. Anxiety and worry use up energy that is needed for healing of tissue during the postoperative period. One or more of the following may cause the patient psychological stress.

(1) Loss of a body part.

(2) Unconsciousness and not knowing or being able to control what is happening.

(3) Pain.

(4) Fear of death.

(5) Separation from family and friends.

(6) The effects of surgery on his lifestyle at home and at work.

(7) Exposure of his body to strangers.

d. Surgical procedures usually combine several classifications and descriptors. For example, a trauma patient may require major, reconstructive, emergency surgery. Regardless of the risk, any surgery that imposes physical and psychological stress is rarely considered "minor" by the patient.

## SECTION I. PREOPERATIVE PATIENT CARE

### 8-3. NURSING IMPLICATIONS

a. Patients are admitted to the health care facility for surgical intervention from a variety of situations and in various physical conditions. The nurse is responsible for completion of preoperative forms, implementing doctor's orders for preoperative care, and documentation of all nursing measures.

b. The following nursing implications are related to preparing a patient for surgery.

(1) Prepare the patient's chart using DD Form 1924, Surgical Check List (figure 8-1). DD Form 1924 contains the following information:

(a) Space for the patient's identification.

(b) A checklist for pertinent clinical records.

(c) A space for recording the most current set of vital signs taken prior to preoperative medications.

(d) A space to indicate allergies.

(e) A space to document all preoperative nursing measures.

(f) A space to document any comment that indicates something very special about this particular patient (for example, removal of prosthesis, patient hard of hearing).

(g) A space for signature of release by the registered nurse when all actions are completed.

(2) Ensure completion of SF 522, Request for Administration of Anesthesia and for Performance of Operations and Other Procedures (figure 8-2).

(a) SF 522 is a legal document, which satisfies requirement of informed consent. A surgical consent form must be signed by the patient before surgery can be performed.

(b) It must be signed by the physician and anesthesiologist to indicate that all risks of surgery and anesthesia have been fully explained to the patient.

| PATIENT'S IDENTIFICATION | | SURGICAL CHECK LIST<br>WARD/ROOM/BED<br>*INSTRUCTIONS: Initial or mark N/A if not applicable* | |
|---|---|---|---|
| CLINICAL RECORDS | | PRE–OP COUNSELING TO PATIENT | |
| SF 515 (2) – TISSUE EXAMINATION | | PRE–OP PREP | |
| SF 516 (3) – OPERATION REPORT | | A.M. CARE | |
| SF 517 (2) – ANESTHESIA | | VALUABLES AND JEWELRY REMOVED *(Wedding Band may be taped in place)* | |
| SF 518 (3) – BLOOD TRANSFUSION _____ UNITS | | HAIRPINS, LIPSTICK, NAILPOLISH REMOVED | |
| SF 522 – OPERATIVE PERMIT *(Signed)* | | DENTURES/BRIDGE REMOVED | |
| HISTORY AND PHYSICAL | | CONTACT LENSES/GLASS EYE, GLASSES, HAIRPIECE, PROSTHESIS REMOVED | |
| SF 511 – T. P. R. GRAPHIC | | VOIDED *(Specify time)* | |
| NURSES NOTES & DOCTORS ORDERS | | ENEMA *(If Ordered)* | |
| X–RAY *(ONLY the required)* | | ID BAND ON ARM | |
| REPORTS | | INPATIENT IDENT PLATE *(In envelope)* | |
| FILMS | | | |
| LABORATORY REPORTS *(ONLY the required)* | | | |
| HEMATOLOGY | | PRE–OP MEDICATION *(Specify kind and time administered)* | |
| URINE | | | |
| EKG | | | |
| | | | |
| TPR AND BP *(Prior to pre-op medication)* | | CATHETER IN PLACE ☐ YES ☐ NO ☐ CLAMPED ☐ TO DRAINAGE | |
| KNOWN ALLERGIES | | | |
| COMMENTS: | | | |
| SIGNATURE OF NURSE RELEASING PATIENT TO OPERATING ROOM | | | |

*FOR INPATIENT IDENTIFICATION PLATE*

**DD FORM 1924**, 1 SEP 73 — REPLACES DA FORM 3629, 1 JUL 72, AND AF FORM 534, SEP 70, WHICH WILL BE USED UNTIL EXHAUSTED.

***PEEL COVER FROM ADHESIVE ON REVERSE SIDE AND FOLD BACK AT DOTTED LINE TO MAKE ENVELOPE FOR PLATE STORAGE***

Figure 8-1. DD Form, 1924, Surgical Check List.

| MEDICAL RECORD | REQUEST FOR ADMINISTRATION OF ANESTHESIA AND FOR PERFORMANCE OF OPERATIONS AND OTHER PROCEDURES |
|---|---|

**A. IDENTIFICATION**

1. OPERATION OR PROCEDURE

**B. STATEMENT OF REQUEST**

1. The nature and purpose of the operation or procedure, possible alternative methods of treatment, the risks involved, and the possibility of complications have been fully explained to me. I acknowledge that no guarantees have been made to me concerning the results of the operation or procedure. I understand the nature of the operation or procedure to be ______________________
*(Description of operation or procedure in layman's language)*

______________________

______________________

which is to be performed by or under the direction of Dr. ______________________

2. I request the performance of the above-named operation or procedure and of such additional operations or procedures as are found to be necessary or desirable, in the judgment of the professional staff of the below-named medical facility, during the course of the above-named operation or procedure.

3. I request the administration of such anesthesia as may be considered necessary or advisable in the judgment of the professional staff of the below-named medical facility.

4. Exceptions to surgery or anesthesia, if any, are: ______________________
*(If "none", so state)*

5. I request the disposal by authorities of the below-named medical facility of any tissues or parts which it may be necessary to remove.

6. I understand that photographs and movies may be taken of this operation, and that they may be viewed by various personnel undergoing training or indoctrination at this or other facilities. I consent to the taking of such pictures and observation of the operation by authorized personnel, subject to the following conditions:

   a. The name of the patient and his/her family is not used to identify said pictures

   b. Said pictures be used only for purposes of medical/dental study or research.

*(Cross out any parts above which are not appropriate)*

**C. SIGNATURES** *(Appropriate items in Parts A and B must be completed before signing)*

1. COUNSELING PHYSICIAN/DENTIST: I have counseled this patient as to the nature of the proposed procedure(s), attendant risks involved, and expected results, as described above.

______________________
(Signature of Counseling Physician/Dentist)

2. PATIENT: I understand the nature of the proposed procedure(s), attendant risks involved, and expected results, as described above, and hereby request such procedure(s) be performed.

| (Signature of Witness, excluding members of operating team) | (Signature of Patient) | (Date and Time) |
|---|---|---|

3. SPONSOR OR GUARDIAN: (When patient is a minor or unable to give consent) I, ______________________ sponsor/guardian of ______________________ understand the nature of the proposed procedure(s), attendant risks involved, and expected results, as described above, and hereby request such procedure(s) be performed.

| (Signature of Witness, excluding members of operating team) | (Signature of Sponsor/Legal Guardian) | (Date and Time) |
|---|---|---|

| PATIENT'S IDENTIFICATION *(For typed or written entries give: Name—last, first, middle; grade; date; hospital or medical facility)* | REGISTER NO. | WARD NO. |
|---|---|---|

STANDARD FORM 522 (Rev. 10–76)
General Services Administration &
Interagency Comm. on Medical Records
FPMR 101-11.806-8
522-109

GPO : 1987 0 - 191-294

NSN 7540-00-634-4165

Figure 8.2. SF 522, Request for Administration of Anesthesia and for Performance of Operations and Other Procedures.

(c) The patient must sign in the presence of a witness, to consent for the surgical procedure. The witness is attesting to the patient's signature, not to the patient's understanding of the surgical risks. If the adult patient is unconscious, semiconscious, or is not mentally competent, the consent form may be signed by a family member or legal guardian.

(d) If the patient is a minor (usually under the age of 18), the consent form is signed by a parent or legal guardian. A minor who lives away from home and is self-supporting is considered emancipated and he may sign.

(e) Legal age is established on a state-by-state basis. Be familiar with the age of consent for the state in which the health care facility is located and with legal implications when a person other than the patient signs the consent form.

(f) Legal consent forms must be signed prior to administration of preoperative medication or any type of mind-altering medication or the document is not legally binding.

(g) SF 522 must be timed and dated.

(3) Implement doctor's orders for preoperative care.

(a) If ordered, administer an enema. The enema cleanses the colon of fecal material, which reduces the possibility of wound contamination during surgery.

(b) If ordered, assure that the operative site skin prep (shave) is done. An operating room technician or other designated person will clean and shave a wide area surrounding the planned site for the incision. (This may be done in the operating room immediately before surgery). The skin prep frees the skin of hair and microorganisms as much as possible, thus decreasing the possibility of them entering the wound via the skin surface during surgery.

(c) The doctor will give specific directions concerning withholding food and fluid before surgery. Assure that the order is followed. Typically, the patient may eat solid food until supper, but can have nothing by mouth (NPO) beginning at midnight before surgery. Place the NPO sign outside the patient's room. Instruct the patient of the importance and the reason for being NPO. Remove the water pitcher and the drinking glass. Clearly mark the diet roster.

(d) If ordered, administer a sedative. The evening before surgery a hypnotic drug, such as flurazepam hydrochloride (Dalmane®) may be given so that the patient can get a good night's sleep.

## 8-4. PREPARING THE PATIENT FOR SURGERY

a. Preoperative preparation may extend over a period of several days. The patient may undergo tests, radiographic studies, and laboratory procedures. A medical history is taken and a physical examination performed before surgery. Patients scheduled for elective surgery may have laboratory tests such as urinalysis, complete blood count, hemoglobin, and hematocrit done as an outpatient. The nurse plays an important role in explaining the necessity for preoperative tests and in carrying out preparations for these tests. The immediate preparation for surgery usually starts the evening before surgery. Nursing implications related to the preoperative preparation of a patient are:

(1) Assist the patient with personal hygiene and related preoperative care.

(a) The evening before surgery, the patient should take a bath or shower, and shampoo hair to remove excess body dirt and oils. The warm water will also help to relax the patient. Sometimes plain soap and water are used for cleansing the skin, but a topical antiseptic may be used.

(b) Remove all makeup and nail polish. Numerous areas (face, lips, oral mucosa, and nail beds) must be observed for evidence of cyanosis. Makeup and nail polish hide true coloration.

(c) Jewelry and other valuables should be removed for safe keeping. The patient may wear a wedding band to surgery, but it must be secured with tape and gauze wrapping. Do not wrap tightly; circulation may be impaired. Do not leave valuables in the bedside stand or store in the narcotics container. If possible, send these items home with a relative until the patient has need of them. Chart what has been done with the valuables.

(2) Provide information concerning surgery.

(a) The patient is told about the risks and benefits of surgery, the likely outcome if surgery is not performed, and alternative methods of treatment by his doctor. However, the nurse can help the patient cope with the upcoming surgery by taking the time to listen to the patient and others who are concerned about his well being, and answering other questions.

(b) Explain each preoperative nursing measure.

(c) Provide an opportunity for the patient to express his feelings. Ask about spiritual needs and whether he wishes to see a Chaplain.

(d) Provide family members with information concerning their role the morning of the surgery. Give them the surgical waiting room location, and the probable time that they can visit the patient after surgery. Explain the rationale for the patient's stay in the recovery room. Inform them of any machines or tubes that may be attached to the patient following surgery.

(3) Provide preoperative morning care.

(a) Awake the patient early enough to complete morning care. Give him a clean hospital gown and the necessary toiletries. The patient should have another shower or bath using a topical antiseptic, such as povidone-iodine. The skin cannot be made completely sterile, but the number of microorganisms on it can be substantially reduced. If the surgery is extensive, it may be several days before the patient has another shower or "real" bath.

(b) The patient should have complete mouth care before surgery. A clean mouth provides comfort for the patient and prevents aspiration of small food particles that may be left in the mouth. Instruct the patient not to chew gum.

(4) Remove prostheses. Assist the patient or provide privacy so that the patient can remove any prostheses. These includes artificial limbs, artificial eyes, contact lenses, eyeglasses, dentures, or other removable oral appliances. Place small items in a container and label them with the patient's name and room number. Dentures are usually left at the bedside.

(5) Record vital signs. Obtain and record the patient's temperature, pulse, respiration, and blood pressure <u>before</u> the preoperative medication is administered.

b. Allow the patient time to complete any last minute personal measures and visit with the family.

c. Recheck the accuracy of DD Form 1924, Surgical Check List.

d. If ordered, administer preoperative medications. Pre-op medications are usually ordered by the anesthesiologist, and administered about 30 to 60 minutes before the patient is taken to the operating room.

(1) The medications may be ordered given at a scheduled time or on call (the operating room will call and tell you when to give the medications).

(2) The medications may consist of one, two, or three drugs: a narcotic or sedative; a drug to decrease secretions in the mouth, nose, throat, and bronchi; and an antiemetic.

(3) Have the patient void before administering the medications.

(4) Explain to the patient the effects experienced following administration of the medications (drowsiness, extreme dry mouth).

(5) Instruct the patient to remain in bed. Raise the side rails on the bed and place the call bell within easy reach.

e. Assist the operating room technician. The patient is usually transported to the operating room on a wheeled litter, or gurney. The technician should cover the patient with a clean sheet or cotton blanket. Assist the technician to position the patient on the litter. See that the patient is comfortable, and that the restraint is fastened to prevent him from falling off the litter.

## 8-5. DOCUMENT NURSING MEASURES

a. All necessary information should be recorded on the chart before the patient leaves the nursing unit. Check the patient's identification band to be sure the right patient is being taken to surgery. Check the consent form to be sure that it is correctly signed and witnessed.

b. "Sign out" the patient in the nurse's notes. Include the date, the time, the event, and your observations on the status of the patient. "Sign off" DD Form 1924, Surgical Check List.

# SECTION II. THE INTRAOPERATIVE PHASE

## 8-6. THE SURGICAL TEAM

a. **Key Members.** The intraoperative phase begins when the patient is received in the surgical area and lasts until the patient is transferred to the recovery area. Although the surgeon has the most important role in this phase, there are five key members of the surgical team.

b. **The Surgeon.** The surgeon is the leader of the surgical team. The surgeon is ultimately responsible for performing the surgery effectively and safely; however, he is dependent upon other members of the team for the patient's emotional well being and physiologic monitoring.

c. **Anesthesiologist/Anesthetist.** An anesthesiologist is a physician trained in the administration of anesthetics. An anesthetist is a registered professional nurse trained to administer anesthetics. The responsibilities of the anesthesiologist or anesthetist include:

(1) Providing a smooth induction of the patient's anesthesia in order to prevent pain.

(2) Maintaining satisfactory degrees of relaxation of the patient for the duration of the surgical procedure.

(3) Continuous monitoring of the physiologic status of the patient for the duration of the surgical procedure.

(4) Continuous monitoring of the physiologic status of the patient to include oxygen exchange, systemic circulation, neurologic status, and vital signs.

(5) Advising the surgeon of impending complications and independently intervening as necessary.

d. **Scrub Nurse/Assistant.** The scrub nurse or scrub assistant is a nurse or surgical technician who prepares the surgical set-up, maintains surgical asepsis while draping and handling instruments, and assists the surgeon by passing instruments, sutures, and supplies. The scrub nurse must have extensive knowledge of all instruments and how they are used. In the Army, the Operating Room Technician (MOS 91D) often fills this role. The scrub nurse or assistant wears sterile gown, cap, mask, and gloves.

e. **Circulating Nurse.** The circulating nurse is a professional registered nurse who is liaison between scrubbed personnel and those outside of the operating room. The circulating nurse is free to respond to request from the surgeon, anesthesiologist or anesthetist, obtain supplies, deliver supplies to the sterile field, and carry out the nursing care plan. The circulating nurse does not scrub or wear sterile gloves or a sterile gown. Other responsibilities include:

(1) Initial assessment of the patient on admission to the operating room, helping onitoring the patient.

(2) Assisting the surgeon and scrub nurse to don sterile gowns and gloves.

(3) Anticipating the need for equipment, instruments, medications, and blood components, opening packages so that the scrub nurse can remove the sterile supplies, preparing labels, and arranging for transfer of specimens to the laboratory for analysis.

(4) Saving all used and discarded gauze sponges, and at the end of the operation, counting the number of sponges, instruments, and needles used during the operation to prevent the accidental loss of an item in the wound.

## 8-7. MAJOR CLASSIFICATIONS OF ANESTHETIC AGENTS

a. There are three major classifications of anesthetic agents: general anesthetic, regional anesthetic, and local anesthetic. A general anesthetic produces loss of consciousness and thus affects the total person. When the patient is given drugs to produce central nervous system depression, it is termed general anesthesia.

(1) There are three phases of general anesthesia: induction, maintenance, and emergence. Induction, (rendering the patient unconscious) begins with administration of the anesthetic agent and continues until the patient is ready for the incision. Maintenance (surgical anesthesia) begins with the initial incision and continues until near completion of the procedure. Emergence begins when the patient starts to come out from under the effects of the anesthesia and usually ends when the patient leaves the operating room. The advantage of general anesthesia is that it can be used for patients of any age and for any surgical procedure, and leave the patient unaware of the physical trauma. The disadvantage is that it carries major risks of circulatory and respiratory depression.

(2) Routes of administration of a general anesthetic agent are rectal (which is not used much in today's medical practices), intravenous infusion, and inhalation. No single anesthetic meets the criteria for an ideal general anesthetic. To obtain optimal effects and decrease likelihood of toxicity, administration of a general anesthetic requires the use of one or more agents. Often an intravenous drug such as thiopental sodium (Pentothal) is used for induction and then supplemented with other agents to produce surgical anesthesia. Inhalation anesthesia is often used because it has the advantage of rapid excretion and reversal of effects.

(3) Characteristics of the ideal general anesthetic are:

(a) It produces analgesia.

(b) It produces complete loss of consciousness.

(c) It provides a degree of muscle relaxation.

(d) It dulls reflexes.

(e) It is safe and has minimal side effects.

(4) General anesthesia is used for major head and neck surgery, intracranial surgery, thoracic surgery, upper abdominal surgery, and surgery of the upper and lower extremities.

b. A regional or block anesthetic agent causes loss of sensation in a large region of the body. The patient remains awake but loses sensation in the specific region anesthetized. In some instances, reflexes are lost also. When an anesthetic agent is injected near a nerve or nerve pathway, it is termed regional anesthesia.

(1) Regional anesthesia may be accomplished by nerve blocks, or subdural or epidural blocks (see figure 8-3).

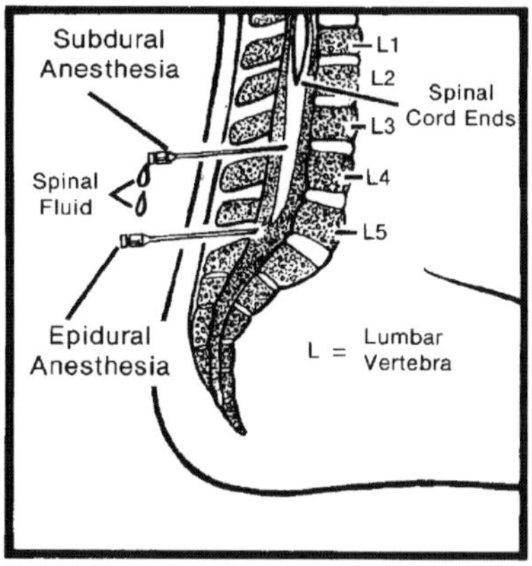


Figure 8-3. Sites for spinal anesthetics.

(2) Nerve blocks are done by injecting a local anesthetic around a nerve trunk supplying the area of surgery such as the jaw, face, and extremities.

(3) Subdural blocks are used to provide spinal anesthesia. The injection of an anesthetic, through a lumbar puncture, into the cerebrospinal fluid in the subarachnoid space causes sensory, motor and autonomic blockage, and is used for surgery of the lower abdomen, perineum, and lower extremities. Side effects of spinal anesthesia include headache, hypotension, and urinary retention.

(4) For epidural block, the agent is injected through the lumbar interspace into the epidural space, that is, outside the spinal canal.

c. Local anesthesia is administration of an anesthetic agent directly into the tissues. It may be applied topically to skin surfaces and the mucous membranes in the nasopharynx, mouth, vagina, or rectum or injected intradermally into the tissue. Local infiltration is used in suturing small wounds and in minor surgical procedures such as skin biopsy. Topical anesthesia is used on mucous membranes, open skin surfaces, wounds, and burns. The advantage of local anesthesia is that it acts quickly and has few side-effects.

## 8-8. SELECTION OF AN ANESTHETIC AGENT

a. Depending on its classification, anesthesia produces states such as narcosis (loss of consciousness), analgesia (insensibility to pain), loss of reflexes, and relaxation. General anesthesia produces all of these responses. Regional anesthesia does not cause narcosis, but does result in analgesia and reflex loss. Local anesthesia results in loss of sensation in a small area of tissue.

b. The choice of route and the type of anesthesia is primarily made by the anesthetist or anesthesiologist after discussion with the patient. Whether by intravenous, inhalation, oral, or rectal route, many factors effect the selection of an anesthetic agent:

(1) The type of surgery.

(2) The location and type of anesthetic agent required.

(3) The anticipated length of the procedure.

(4) The patient's condition.

(5) The patient's age.

(6) The patient's previous experiences with anesthesia.

(7) The available equipment.

(8) Preferences of the anesthesiologist or anesthetist and the patient.

(9) The skill of the anesthesiologist or anesthetist.

c. Factors considered by the anesthetist or anesthesiologist when selecting an agent are the smoking and drinking habits of the patient, any medications the patient is taking, and the presence of disease. Of particular concern are pulmonary function, hepatic function, renal function, and cardiovascular function.

(1) Pulmonary function is adversely affected by upper respiratory tract infections and chronic obstructive lung diseases such as emphysema, especially when intensified by the effects of general anesthesia. These conditions also predispose the patient to postoperative lung infections.

(2) Liver diseases such as cirrhosis impair the ability of the liver to detoxify medications used during surgery, to produce the prothrombin necessary for blood clotting, and to metabolize nutrients essential for healing following surgery.

(3) Renal insufficiency may alter the excretion of drugs and influence the patient's response to the anesthesia. Regulation of fluids and electrolytes, as well as acid-base balance, may be impaired by renal disease.

(4) Well-controlled cardiac conditions pose minimal surgical risks. Severe hypertension, congestive heart failure, or recent myocardial infarction drastically increase the risks.

d. Medications, whether prescribed or over-the-counter, can affect the patient's reaction to the anesthetic agent, increase the effects of the anesthesia, and increase the risk from the stress of surgery. Medication is usually withheld when the patient goes to surgery; but some specific medications are given even then. For example, patients with cardiovascular problems or diabetes mellitus may continue to receive their prescribed medications.

(1) Because some medications interact adversely with other medications and with anesthetic agents, preoperative assessment should include a thorough medication history. Patients may be taking medication for conditions unrelated to the surgery, and are unaware of the potential for adverse reactions of these medications with anesthetic agents.

(2) Drugs in the following categories increase surgical risk.

(a) Adrenal steroids--abrupt withdrawal may cause cardiovascular collapse in long-term users.

(b) Antibiotics--may be incompatible with anesthetic agent, resulting in untoward reactions. Those in mycin group may cause respiratory paralysis when combined with certain muscle relaxants used during surgery.

(c) Anticoagulants--may precipitate hemorrhage.

(d) Diuretics--may cause electrolyte (especially potassium) imbalances, resulting in respiratory depression from the anesthesia.

(e) Tranquilizers--may increase the hypotensive effect of the anesthetic agent, thus contributing to shock.

## 8-9. REASONS FOR SURGICAL INTERVENTION

Descriptors used to classify surgical procedures include ablative, diagnostic, constructive, reconstructive, palliative, and transplant. These descriptors are directly related to the reasons for surgical intervention:

a. To cure an illness or disease by removing the diseased tissue or organs.

b. To visualize internal structures during diagnosis.

c. To obtain tissue for examination.

d. To prevent disease or injury.

e. To improve appearance.

f. To repair or remove traumatized tissue and structures.

g. To relieve symptoms or pain.

# SECTION III. RECOVERY ROOM CARE

## 8-10. THE RECOVERY ROOM

a. The recovery room is defined as a specific nursing unit, which accommodates patients who have undergone major or minor surgery. Following the operation, the patient is carefully moved from the operating table to a wheeled stretcher or bed and transferred to the recovery room. The patient usually remains in the recovery room until he begins to respond to stimuli. General nursing goals of care for a patient in the recovery room are:

(1) <u>To support the patient through his state of dependence to independence</u>. Surgery traumatizes the body, decreasing its energy and resistance. Anesthesia impairs the patient's ability to respond to environmental stimuli and to help himself. An artificial airway is usually maintained in place until reflexes for gagging and swallowing return.

When the reflexes return, the patient usually spits out the airway. Position the unconscious patient with his head to the side and slightly down. This position keeps the tongue forward, preventing it from blocking the throat and allows mucus or vomitus to drain out of the mouth rather than down the respiratory tree. Do not place a pillow under the head during the immediate postanesthetic stage. *Patients who have had spinal anesthetics usually lie flat for 8 to 12 hours.* The return of reflexes indicates that anesthesia is ending. Call the patient by name in a normal tone of voice and tell him repeatedly that the surgery is over and that he is in the recovery room.

(2) To relieve the patient's discomfort. Pain is usually greatest for 12 to 36 hours after surgery, decreasing on the second and third post-op day. Analgesics are usually administered every 4 hours the first day. Tension increases pain perception and responses, thus analgesics are most effective if given before the patient's pain becomes severe. Analgesics may be administered in patient controlled infusions.

(3) Early detection of complications. Most people recover from surgery without incident. Complications or problems are relatively rare, but the recovery room nurse must be aware of the possibility and clinical signs of complications.

(4) Prevention of complications. Complications that should be prevented in the recovery room are respiratory distress and hypovolemic shock.

b. The difference between the recovery room and surgical intensive care are:

(1) The recovery room staff supports patients for a few hours until they have recovered from anesthesia.

(2) The surgical intensive care staff supports patients for a prolonged stay, which may last 24 hours or longer.

## 8-11. RESPIRATORY DISTRESS

a. Respiratory distress is the most common recovery room emergency. It may be caused by laryngospasm, aspiration of vomitus, or depressed respirations resulting from medications.

(1) A laryngospasm is a sudden, violent contraction of the vocal cords; a complication, which may happen after the patient's endotracheal tube, is removed. During the surgical procedure with general anesthesia, an endotracheal tube is inserted to maintain patent air passages. The endotracheal tube may be connected to a mechanical ventilator. Upon completion of the operation, the endotracheal tube is removed by the anesthesiologist or anesthetist and replaced by an oropharyngeal airway (figure 8-4).

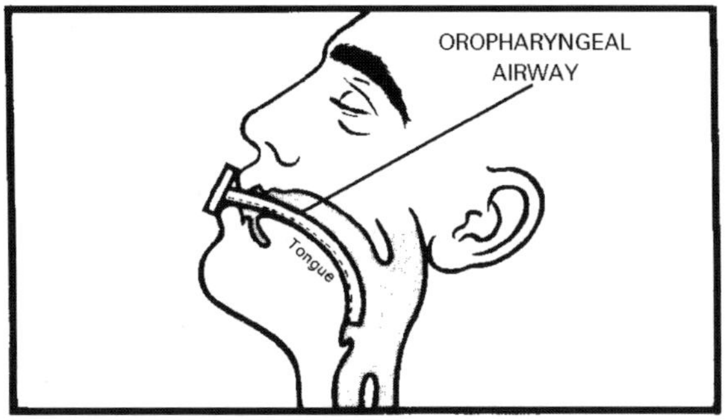


Figure 8-4. Oropharyngeal airway.

(2) Swallowing and cough reflexes are diminished by the effects of anesthesia and secretions are retained. To prevent aspiration, vomitus or secretions should be removed promptly by suction.

(3) Ineffective airway clearance may be related to the effects of anesthesia and drugs that were administered before and during surgery. If possible, an unconscious or semiconscious patient should be placed in a position that allows fluids to drain from the mouth.

b. After removal of the endotracheal tube by the anesthesiologist or anesthetist, an oropharyngeal airway is inserted to prevent the tongue from obstructing the passage of air during recovery from anesthesia. The airway is left in place until the patient is conscious.

## 8-12. PREVENTION OF RESPIRATORY DISTRESS

a. Monitor respiratory status as frequently as prescribed. Respiratory function is assessed by monitoring the patient's respiratory rate, rhythm, and depth, and by observing skin color. The following observations indicate ineffective ventilation:

(1) Restlessness and apprehension.

(2) Unequal chest expansion with use of accessory muscles.

(3) Shallow, noisy respirations.

(4) Cyanosis.

(5) Rapid pulse rate.

b. Report labored respirations to supervisor.

c. Report shallow, rapid respirations to the supervisor.

d. Maintain a patent airway with or without an oropharyngeal tube.

e. Maintain the patient in a position to facilitate lung expansion, usually in Fowler's position.

f. Administer oxygen as ordered.

g. Prevent aspiration of vomitus.

(1) Maintain the position of the patient's head to one side and place an emesis basin under the cheek, extending from just below the eye to the lower edge of the bottom lip.

(2) Wipe vomitus or secretions from the nose or mouth in order to avoid possible aspiration of these fluids into the lungs.

h. Suction the patient either through the nose or mouth as ordered.

## 8-13. HYPOVOLEMIC SHOCK

a. When there is an alteration in circulatory control or a loss of circulating fluid, the body's reaction is shock. The most common type of shock seen in the postoperative patient is ***hypovolemic shock,*** which occurs with a decrease in blood volume. Common signs and symptoms are hypotension; cold, clammy skin; a weak, thready, and rapid pulse; deep, rapid respirations; decreased urine output; thirst; apprehension; and restlessness.

b. Hemorrhage, which is an excessive blood loss, may lead to hypovolemic shock. Postoperative hemorrhage may occur from a slipped suture, a dislodged clot in a wound, or stress on the operative site. It also may result from the pathological disorder for which the patient is being treated, or be caused by certain medications.

c. The primary nursing care goal is to maintain tissue perfusion by eliminating the cause of the shock.

(1) The blood loss from surgery that causes hypovolemic shock may be internal or external.

(2) The loss of fluid or blood volume does not have to be rapid or copious amounts to cause shock.

d. The primary purposes of care for the patient having a hemorrhage include stopping the bleeding and replacing blood volume.

## 8-14. DETECTION OF PENDING HYPOVOLEMIC SHOCK

a. Inspect the surgical dressing frequently and report any bleeding to the supervisor. Also inspect the bedding beneath the patient because blood may drain down the sides of a large dressing and pool under the patient. When reporting bleeding, note the color of the blood. Bright red blood signifies fresh bleeding. Dark, brownish blood indicates that the bleeding is not fresh.

b. Outline the perimeter of the blood stain on the original dressing. Reinforce the original dressing, and make note on the dressing of the date and time the outline was made.

c. Document your observations and the action taken in the nurse's notes.

d. Monitor the patient's vital signs as ordered and report any of the following abnormalities to the supervisor.

(1) A drop in blood pressure (systolic reading below 90 in an adult indicates possible shock; systolic below 80 means actual shock).

(2) A rapid, weak pulse.

(3) Restlessness.

(4) Cool, moist, pale skin.

(5) Tingling of the lips.

(6) Pallor or blueness (cyanosis) of the lips, nailbeds, or conjunctiva (a dark-skinned persons lips will appear a dusky gray).

e. Administer narcotics only after checking doctor's orders and consulting with supervisor. If shock is imminent, it may be precipitated by administration of narcotics.

f. Administer fluids to replace volume in accordance with the doctor's orders. The doctor may order that blood volume be replaced by intravenous (IV) fluids, plasma expanders, or whole blood products.

## 8-15. GENERAL NURSING CARE OF A PATIENT IN THE RECOVERY ROOM

a. When the patient is moved to the recovery room, every effort should be made to avoid unnecessary strain, exposure, or possible injury. The anesthesiologist or anesthetist goes to the recovery room with the patient, reports his condition, leaves postoperative orders and any special instructions, and monitors his condition until that responsibility is transferred to the recovery room nurses. The recovery room nurse should check the doctor's orders and carry them out immediately.

b. Patients are concentrated in a limited area to make it possible for one nurse to give close attention to two or three patients at the same time. Each patient unit has a recovery bed equipped with side rails, poles for IV medications, and a chart rack. The bed is easily moved and adjusted. Each unit has outlets for piped-in oxygen, suction, and blood pressure apparatus. The following are nursing implications for the general care of a patient in the recovery room:

(1) Maintain proper functioning of drains, tubes, and intravenous infusions. Prevent kinking or clogging that interferes with adequate flow of drainage through catheters and drainage tubes.

(2) Monitor intake and output precisely, to include all Intravenous fluids and blood products, urine, vomitus, nasogastric tube drainage, and wound drainage.

(3) Observe and document the patient's level of consciousness. The return of central nervous system function is assessed through response to stimuli and orientation. Levels of consciousness return in reverse order: unconscious, responds to touch and sound, drowsy, awake but not oriented, and awake and oriented. Specific criteria is usually used for categorizing the recovery room patient.

(a) Comatose -- unconscious; unresponsive to stimuli.

(b) Stupor -- lethargic and unresponsive; unaware of surroundings.

(c) Drowsy -- half asleep, sluggish; responds to touch and sounds.

(d) Alert -- able to give appropriate response to stimuli.

(4) Implement safety measures to protect the patient. Keep the side rails raised at all times. Assure that the patient is positioned so that he is not tangled in or laying on IV or drainage tubes. Do not use a head pillow while the patient is unconscious, or for eight hours if the patient had spinal anesthesia. Turn the patient's head to one side when he is in the supine position so that secretions can drain from the mouth and the tongue will not fall into the throat to block the air passage. When the patient is alert, show him how to use the call bell and place it where it is readily available.

(5) If the patient had a spinal anesthetic, observe and report any feeling or spontaneous movement. Movement usually returns before feeling. Movement returns in the patient's toes first, and moves upward. As the anesthesia wears off, the patient will begin to have sensation often described as "pins and needles." Spinal anesthesia wears off slowly. Keep the patient in a supine position for six to eight hours to prevent spinal headache. Turn the patient from side to side and prop up with pillows for a few minutes to relieve pressure on the back, but only if permitted by the doctor.

(6) Prevent nosocomial infections. Wash your hands before and after working with each patient. Maintain aseptic technique for incisional wounds. Turn the patient

frequently to prevent respiratory infections. When the patient is alert, encourage and assist him to cough and take deep breaths several times each hour.

(7) If possible, engage the patient in a conversation to observe his level of orientation. Take into consideration each patient's normal responses due to various physical factors.

(8) Provide emotional support to the patient and his family. When the patient is alert, tell him that he is in the recovery room and that you are always nearby to help him. Reinforce any information that may have been provided by the surgeon. To decrease anxiety and increase lung expansion, encourage conversation with the patient. Use this opportunity to patient teach by explaining what you are about to do in brief, simple sentences. If family members are permitted in the recovery room, stay with them as they visit. They may be frightened of the environment and by their loved one's appearance.

(9) When the patient's physical status and level of consciousness are stable, the surgeon clears the patient for transfer to his room. Call the nursing unit and give a verbal report to include the following.

(a) Patient's name

(b) Type of surgery.

(c) Mental alertness.

(d) Care given in the recovery room.

(e) Vital signs, at what time they were taken, and any symptoms of complications.

(f) Presence, type and functional status of intravenous fluids, and any suction or drainage systems.

(g) Whether or not the patient has voided, if a catheter is not in place.

(h) Any medications given in the recovery room.

(10) Document all necessary information in the nurse's notes and transfer the patient to the unit in accordance with local standing operating procedures (SOP).

## SECTION IV. POSTOPERATIVE PATIENT CARE

### 8-16. RECEIVING THE POST-OP PATIENT

a. The nursing process is used during all phases of perioperative care, with emphasis on the special and unique needs of each patient in each phase. Ongoing postoperative care is planned to ease the patient's recovery from surgery. The nursing care plan includes promoting physical and psychological health, preventing complications, and teaching self-care for the patient's return home. While the patient is in the operating and recovery room, an unoccupied bed is prepared. The top linen is folded to the side or bottom of the bed. Absorbent pads are placed over the drawsheet to protect bottom linens. Equipment and supplies, such as blood pressure apparatus, tissues, an emesis basin, and a pole for hanging the intravenous fluid containers, should be in place when the patient returns. The unit nurse should be informed by the recovery room nurse if other items, such as suction or oxygen equipment will be needed.

b. Postoperative patient care begins with the unit nurse assisting recovery room personnel in transferring the patient to the bed in his room. Data from the preoperative and intraoperative phases is used to make an initial assessment. The assessment is often combined with implementation of the doctor's postoperative orders and should include the following.

(1) Position and safety. Place the patient in the position ordered by the doctor. The patient who has had spinal anesthesia may have to remain lying flat for several hours. If the patient is not fully conscious, place him in a side-lying position and raise the side rails.

(2) Vital signs. Take vital signs and note alterations from postoperative and recovery room data, as well as any symptoms of complications.

(3) Level of consciousness. Assess the patient's reaction to stimuli and ability to move extremities. Help the patient become oriented by telling him that his surgery is over and that he is back in his room.

(4) Intravenous fluids. Assess the type and amount of solution, the tubing, and the infusion site. Count the rate at which the intravenous fluid is infusing.

(5) Wound. Check the patient's dressing for drainage. Note the color and amount, if any. If there is a large amount of drainage or bright red bleeding, report this immediately to the supervisor.

(6) Drains and tubes. Assess indwelling urinary catheter, gastrointestinal suction, and other tubes for drainage, patency, and amount of output. Be sure drainage bags are hanging properly and suction is functioning. If the patient is receiving oxygen, be sure that the application and flow rate is as ordered.

(7) Color and temperature of skin. Feel the patient's skin for warmth and perspiration. Observe the patient for paleness or cyanosis.

(8) Comfort. Assess the patient for pain, nausea, and vomiting. If the patient has pain, note the location, duration and intensity. Determine from recovery room data if analgesics were given and at what time.

c. Make sure that the patient is warm and comfortable, and allow family members to visit after you have completed the initial assessment.

## 8-17. THE EFFECTS OF ANESTHESIA

a. The effects of anesthesia tend to last well into the postoperative period. Anesthetic agents may depress respiratory function, cardiac output, peristalsis and normal functioning of the gastrointestinal tract, and may temporarily depress bladder tone and response.

(1) Effects on the respiratory system. Pulmonary efficiency is reduced, increasing the possibility of postoperative pneumonia. *Pneumonia* is an inflammation of the alveoli resulting from an infectious process or the presence of foreign material. Pneumonia can occur postoperatively because of aspiration, infection, depressed cough reflex, immobilization, dehydration, or increased secretions from anesthesia. Signs and symptoms common to pneumonia are an elevated temperature, chills, cough producing purulent or rusty sputum, dyspnea, and chest pain. The purposes of medical intervention is to treat the underlying infection, maintain respiratory status, and prevent the spread of infection.

(2) Effects on the cardiovascular system. Anesthesia may affect cardiac output, thus increasing the possibility of unstable blood pressure. Shock is the reaction to acute peripheral circulatory failure because of an alteration in circulatory control or to a loss of circulating fluid.

(3) Effects on the urinary system. Anesthesia can cause urinary retention. Decreased fluid intake can lead to dehydration. Assess urinary elimination status by measuring intake and output. Offer the bedpan or urinal at regular intervals to promote voiding. If catheter is present, monitor drainage.

(4) Effects on gastrointestinal system. Anesthesia slows or stops the peristaltic action of the intestines resulting in constipation, abdominal distention, and flatulence. Anesthesia may also cause nausea and vomiting resulting in a fluid imbalance. Ordinarily, intravenous infusions are used while the patient takes nothing by mouth until bowel sounds are heard upon auscultation. Observe the patient for abdominal distention. Have the patient move about in bed and walk to help promote the movement and expulsion of the flatus.

b. A wide variety of factors increase the risk of postoperative complications. Comfort is often the priority for the patient following surgery. Nausea, vomiting, and other effects of anesthesia cause alterations in comfort. The nursing care plan should include activities to meet the patient's needs while helping him cope with these alterations.

## 8-18. OTHER POSTOPERATIVE COMPLICATIONS

a. ***Atelectasis*** is the incomplete expansion or collapse of alveoli with retained mucus, involving a portion of the lung and resulting in poor gas exchange. Signs and symptoms of atelectasis include dyspnea, cyanosis, restlessness, apprehension, crackles, and decreased lung sounds over affected areas. The primary purposes of care for the patient with atelectasis are to ensure oxygenation of tissue, prevent further atelectasis, and expand the involved lung tissue.

b. ***Hypovolemic shock*** is the type most commonly seen in the postoperative patient. Hypovolemic shock occurs when there is a decrease in blood volume. Signs and symptoms are hypotension; cold, clammy skin; a weak, thready and rapid pulse; deep, rapid respirations; decreased urine output; thirst; restlessness; and apprehension.

c. ***Hemorrhage*** is excessive blood loss, either internally or externally. Hemorrhage may lead to hypovolemic shock.

d. ***Thrombophlebitis*** is inflammation of a vein associated with thrombus (blood clot) formation. Thrombophlebitis is more commonly seen in the legs of a postoperative patient. Signs and symptoms are elevated temperature, pain and cramping in the calf or thigh of the involved extremity, redness and swelling in the affected area, and pain with dorsiflexion of the foot (figure 8-5). Care for the patient with thrombophlebitis includes preventing a clot from breaking loose and becoming an embolus that travels to the lungs, heart, or brain and preventing other clot formation.

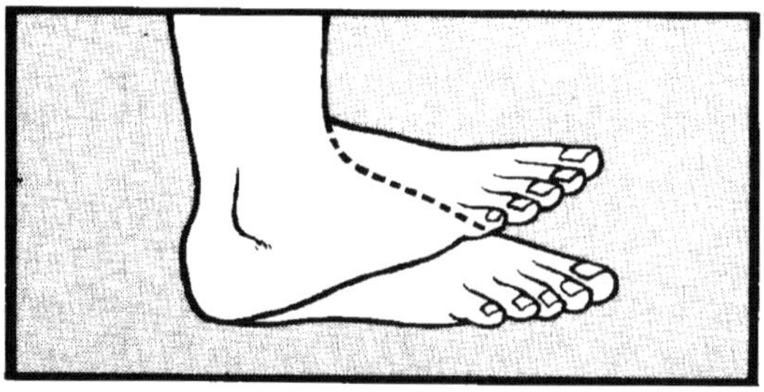

Figure 8-5. Dorsiflection of the foot.

## 8-19. WOUND COMPLICATIONS

a. Nursing implications in relation to prevention and early detection of wound complications include assessing vital signs, especially monitoring an elevated temperature; assisting the patient to maintain nutritional status, and use of medical asepsis. The integumentary system is the body's natural barrier against invasion of infectious microorganisms. Possible negative effects of surgery on the integumentary system include wound infection, dehiscence, and evisceration.

(1) Wound infection. Surgical wounds are assessed for possible complications by inspection (sight and smell) and palpation for appearance, drainage, and pain. The wound edges should be clean and well approximated with a crust along the wound edges. If infection is present, the wound is slightly swollen, reddened, and feels hot. Hand washing is the most frequently used medical aseptic practice and the single most effective way to prevent the spread of microorganisms that cause wound infections.

(2) Dehiscence. Dehiscence is the separation of wound edges without the protrusion of organs. An appreciable increase in serosanguineous fluid on the wound dressing (usually between the 6th and 8th postoperative day) is a clue to impending dehiscence.

(3) Evisceration. Evisceration is the separation of wound edges with the protrusion of organs through the incision. Wound disruption is often preceded by sudden straining. The patient may feel that something "gave way."

b. If dehiscence is suspected or occurs, place the patient on complete bed rest in a position that puts the least strain on the operative area and notify the surgeon. If evisceration occurs, cover the wound area with sterile towels soaked in saline solution and notify the surgeon immediately. These are both emergency situations that require prompt surgical repair.

c. Predisposing factors and causes of wound separation are:

(1) Infection.

(2) Malnutrition , particularly insufficient protein and vitamin C, which interferes with the normal healing process.

(3) Defective suturing or allergic reaction to the suture material.

(4) Unusual strain on the wound from severe vomiting, coughing, or sneezing.

(5) Extreme obesity, an enlarged abdomen, or an abdomen weakened by prior surgeries may also contribute to the occurrence of wound dehiscence and evisceration.

## 8-20. WOUND CLOSURES AND HEALING

a. Any wound or injury results in repair to the damaged skin and underlying structures. All wounds follow the same phases in healing, although differences occur in the length of time required for each phase of the healing process and in the extent of granulation tissue formed. Wounds heal by one of three processes: primary, secondary, or tertiary intention.

(1) ***Primary intention*** is the ideal method of wound healing. The wound is a clean, straight line with little loss of tissue. All wound edges are well approximated and sutured closed. It is a form of connective tissue repair that involves proliferation of fibroblasts and capillary buds and the subsequent development of collagen to produce a scar. Most surgical incisions and small sutured lacerations heal by primary intention. These wounds normally heal rapidly with minimal scarring.

(2) ***Secondary intention*** is healing of an open wound where there has been a significant loss of tissue. The edges may be so far apart that they cannot be pulled together satisfactorily. Infection may also cause a separation of tissue surfaces and prevent wound approximation. The wound is usually not sutured closed. Granulation tissue is allowed to form, followed by a large scar formation. Epithelium ultimately grows over the scar tissue.

(3) ***Tertiary intention*** is delayed primary closure. The wound is left open for several days and is then sutured closed. There is increased risk of infection and inflammatory reaction. The wound is usually one that is fairly deep and likely to contain accumulating fluid. A drain or pack gauze may be placed into the wound to provide for drainage.

b. The greater the tissue damage, the greater the demand on the body's reparative processes. The ability to close an open wound affects the rate of healing and prevention of complications.

## 8-21. FACTORS WHICH MAY IMPAIR WOUND HEALING

a. **Developmental Stage.** Children and adults in good health heal more rapidly than do elderly persons who have undergone physiologic changes that result in diminished fibroblastic activity and diminished circulation. Older adults are more likely to have chronic illnesses that cause pathologic changes that may impair wound healing.

b. **Poor Circulation and Oxygenation.** Blood supply to the affected area may be diminished in elderly persons and in those with peripheral vascular disorders, cardiovascular disorders, hypertension, or diabetes mellitus. Oxygenation of tissues is decreased in persons who smoke, and in those with anemia or respiratory disorders. Obesity slows wound healing because of the presence of large amounts of fat, which has fewer blood vessels.

c. **Physical and Emotional Wellness.** Chronic physical illness and severe emotional stress have a negative affect on wound healing. Patients who have inadequate nutrition, those who are taking steroid drugs, and those who are receiving postoperative radiation therapy have a higher risk of wound complications and impaired wound healing.

d. **Condition of the Wound.** The specific condition of the wound affects the healing process. Wounds that are infected or contain foreign bodies (including drains, pack gauze) heal slowly.

## 8-22. WOUND DRAINS

a. **Inserting Drains**. The use of drains, tubes, and suction devices at the wound site is often necessary to promote healing. A drain or tube is inserted into or near a wound after the surgical procedure is completed. One end of a tube or drain is placed in or near the incision when it is anticipated that fluid will collect in the closed area and delay healing. The other tube end is passed through the incision or through a separate opening called a stab wound. Tubes that are to be connected to suction or have a built-in reservoir are sutured to the skin. It is important that you know the type of drain or tube in use so that patency and placement can be accurately assessed.

b. **Penrose Drain** (figure 8-6). This is the most commonly used drain. It is made of flexible, soft rubber and causes little tissue reaction. It acts by drawing any pus or fluid along its surfaces through the incision or through a stab wound adjacent to the main incision. It has a large safety pin outside the wound to maintain its position. To facilitate drainage and healing of tissues from the inside to the outside, the tube is often pulled out and shortened 1 to 2 inches each day until it falls out. The safety pin should be placed in its new position prior to cutting the drain. Advance the drain with a dressing forceps or hemostat, use surgical scissors to cut excess drain.

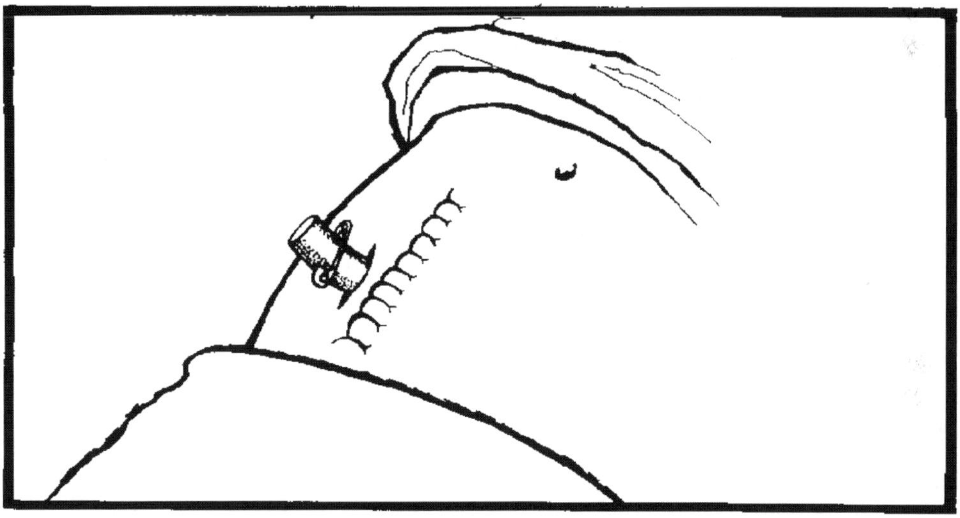

Figure 8-6. Penrose drain.

c. **Jackson-Pratt/Hemovac Closed Suction Device** (figure 8-7). Tubes are connected to suction or there is a built-in reservoir to maintain constant low suction. In the operating room, the surgeon places the perforated drainage tubing in the desired area, makes a stab wound, then draws the excess tubing through the wound creating a tightly sealed porthole. The tubing is then attached via an adaptor to the suction device. To establish negative pressure, compress the device and place the plug in the air hole.

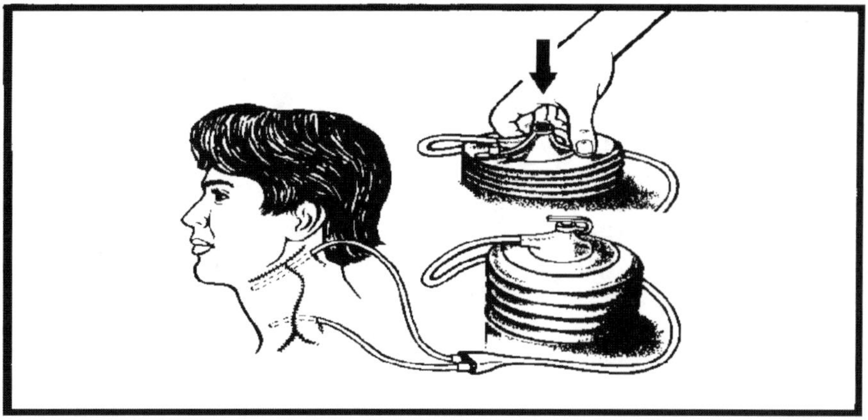

Figure 8-7. Closed suction device.

## 8-23. POSTOPERATIVE PATIENT CARE ACCORDING TO BODY SYSTEM

a. **Respiratory System.** The cough reflex is suppressed during surgery and mucous accumulates in the trachea and bronchi. After surgery, respiration is less effective because of the anesthesia and pain medication, and because deep respirations cause pain at the incision site. As a result, the alveoli do not inflate and may collapse, and retained secretions increase the potential for respiratory infection and atelectasis.

(1) Turn the patient as ordered.

(2) Ambulate the patient as ordered.

(3) If permitted, place the patient in a semi-Fowler's position, with support for the neck and shoulders, to aid lung expansion.

(4) Reinforce the deep breathing exercises the patient was taught preoperatively. Deep breathing exercises hyperventilate the alveoli and prevent their collapse, improve lung expansion and volume, help to expel anesthetic gases and mucus, and facilitate oxygenation of tissues. Ask the patient to:

(a) Exhale gently and completely.

(b) Inhale through the nose gently and completely.

(c) Hold his breath and mentally count to three.

(d) Exhale as completely as possible through pursed lips as if to whistle.

(e) Repeat these steps three times every hour while awake.

(5) Coughing, in conjunction with deep breathing, helps to remove retained mucus from the respiratory tract. Coughing is painful for the postoperative patient. While in a semi-Fowler's position, the patient should support the incision with a pillow or folded bath blanket and follow these guidelines for effective coughing:

(a) Inhale and exhale deeply and slowly through the nose three times.

(b) Take a deep breath and hold it for 3 seconds.

(c) Give two or three "hacking" coughs while exhaling with the mouth open and the tongue out.

(d) Take a deep breath with the mouth open.

(e) Cough deeply once or twice.

(f) Take another deep breath.

(g) Repeat these steps every 2 hours while awake.

(6) An incentive spirometer may be ordered to help increase lung volume, inflation of alveoli, and facilitate venous return. Most patients learn to use this device and can carry out the procedure without a nurse in attendance. Monitor the patient from time to time to motivate them to use the spirometer and to be sure that they use it correctly.

(a) While in an upright position, the patient should take two or three normal breaths, then insert the spirometer's mouthpiece into his mouth.

(b) Inhale through the mouth and hold the breath for 3 to 5 seconds.

(c) Exhale slowly and fully.

(d) Repeat this sequence 10 times during each waking hour for the first 5 post-op days. Do not use the spirometer immediately before or after meals.

b. **Cardiovascular System.** Venous return from the legs slows during surgery and may actually decrease in some surgical positions. With circulatory stasis of the legs, thrombophlebitis and emboli are potential complications of surgery. Venous return is increased by flexion and contraction of the leg muscles.

(1) To prevent thrombophlebitis, instruct the patient to exercise the legs while on bedrest. Leg exercises are easier if the patient is in a supine position with the head of the bed slightly raised to relax abdominal muscles. Leg exercises (figure 8-8) should be individualized using the following guidelines.

(a) Flex and extend the knees, pressing the backs of the knees down toward the mattress on extension.

(b) Alternately, point the toes toward the chin (dorsiflex) and toward the foot of the bed (plantar flex); then, make a circle with the toes.

(c) Raise and lower each leg, keeping the leg straight.

(d) Repeat leg exercises every 1 to 2 hours.

(2) Ambulate the patient as ordered.

(a) Provide physical support for the first attempts.

(b) Have the patient dangle the legs at the bedside before ambulation.

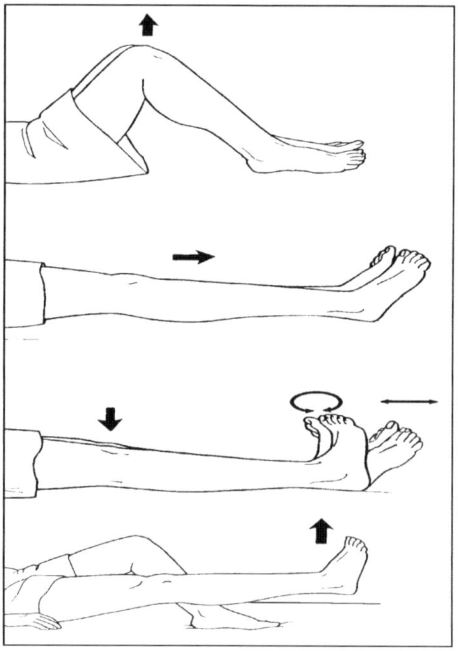

Figure 8-8. Leg exercises.

(c) Monitor the patient's blood pressure while he dangles.

(d) If the patient is hypotensive or experiences dizziness while dangling, do not ambulate. Report this event to the supervisor.

c. **Urinary System.** Patients who have had abdominal surgery, particularly in the lower abdominal and pelvic regions, often have difficulty urinating after surgery. The sensation of needing to urinate may temporarily decrease from operative trauma in the region near the bladder. The fear of pain may cause the patient to feel tense and have difficulty urinating.

(1) If the patient does not have a catheter, and has not voided within eight hours after return to the nursing unit, report this event to the supervisor.

(2) Palpate the patient's bladder for distention and assess the patient's response. The area over the bladder may feel rounder and slightly cooler than the rest of the abdomen. The patient may tell you that he feels a sense of fullness and urgency.

(3) Assist the patient to void.

(a) Assist the patient to the bathroom or provide privacy.

(b) Position the patient comfortably on the bedpan or offer the urinal.

(4) Measure and record urine output. If the first urine voided following surgery is less than 30 cc, notify the supervisor.

(5) If there is blood or other abnormal content in the urine, or the patient complains of pain when voiding, report this to the supervisor.

(6) Follow nursing unit standing operating procedures (SOP) for infection control, when caring for the patient with a Foley catheter.

d. **Gastrointestinal System.** Inactivity and altered fluid and food intake during the perioperative period alter gastrointestinal activities. Nausea and vomiting may result from an accumulation of stomach contents before peristalsis returns or from manipulation of organs during the surgical procedure if the patient had abdominal surgery.

(1) Report to the supervisor if the patient complains of abdominal distention.

(2) Ask the patient if he has passed gas since returning from surgery.

(3) Auscultate for bowel sounds. Report your assessment to the supervisor, and document in nursing notes.

(4) Assess abdominal distention, especially if bowel sounds are not audible or are high-pitched, indicating an absence of peristalsis.

(5) Provide a privacy so that the patient will feel comfortable expelling gas.

(6) Encourage food and fluid intake when the patient in no longer NPO.

(7) Ambulate the patient to assist peristalsis and help relieve gas pain, which is a common postoperative discomfort.

(8) Instruct the patient to tell you of his first bowel movement following surgery. Record the bowel movement on the intake and output (I&O) sheet.

(9) If nursing measures are not effective, the doctor may order medication or an enema to facilitate peristalsis and relieve distention. A last measure may require the insertion of a nasogastric or rectal tube.

(10) Document nursing measures and the results in the nursing notes.

e. **Integumentary System.** Follow doctor's orders for wound care, wound irrigations and cultures. In addition to assessment of the surgical wound, you should evaluate the patient's general condition and laboratory test results. If the patient complains of increased or constant pain from the wound, or if wound edges are swollen or there is purulent drainage, further assessment should be made and your findings reported and documented. Generalized malaise, increased pain, anorexia, and an elevated body temperature and pulse rate are indicators of infection. Important laboratory data include an elevated white blood cell count and the causative organism if a wound culture is done. Staples or sutures are usually removed by the doctor using sterile technique. After the staples or sutures are removed, the doctor may apply Steri-Strip® to the wound to give support as it continues to heal.

(1) There are two methods of caring for wounds: the open method, in which no dressing is used to cover the wound, and the closed method, in which a dressing is applied. The basic objective of wound care is to promote tissue repair and regeneration, so that skin integrity is restores. Dressings have advantages and disadvantages.

(a) Advantages. Dressings absorb drainage, protect the wound from injury and contamination, and provide physical, psychological, and aesthetic comfort for the patient.

(b) Disadvantages. Dressings can rub or stick to the wound, causing superficial injury. Dressings create a warm, damp, and dark environment conducive to the growth of organisms and resultant infection.

(2) At some time, most wounds are covered with a dressing and you may be responsible for changing the dressing. First, gather needed supplies. Items may be packaged individually or all necessary items may be in a sterile dressing tray. Some surgical units have special dressing carts, with agents needed to clean the wound, and materials to cover and secure the dressing. Next, prepare the patient for the dressing change by explaining what will be done, providing privacy for the procedure, and assisting the patient to a position that is comfortable for him and for you. Finally, use appropriate aseptic techniques when changing the dressing and follow precautions for contact with blood and body fluids. The most common cause of nosocomial infections is carelessness

in observing medical and surgical asepsis when changing dressings. It is especially important to wash hands thoroughly before and after changing dressings and to follow the Centers for Disease Control (CDC) guidelines (figure 8-9).

**Precautions for Contact with Blood and Body Fluids**

Wear gloves when touching blood, body fluids containing visible blood, an open wound, or non-intact skin of all clients and when handling items or surfaces soiled with blood or body fluids.

Wash hands thoroughly after removing gloves and if contaminated with blood or with body fluids that contain visible blood.

Take precautions to prevent injuries by needles, sharp instruments, or sharp devices.

Do not give direct client care if you have open or weeping lesions or dermatitis.

If procedures commonly cause droplets or splashing of blood or body fluids to which standard precautions apply, wear gloves, a surgical mask, and protective eyewear, as appropriate.

Figure 8-9. Guidelines.

## 8-24. GENERAL POSTOPERATIVE NURSING IMPLICATIONS

a. Monitor vital signs as ordered.

b. Report elevated temperature and rapid/weak pulse immediately to supervisor (infection).

c. Report lowered blood pressure and increased pulse to supervisor (hypovolemic shock).

d. Administer analgesics as ordered.

e. Apply all nursing implications related to the patient receiving analgesics whether narcotic or nonnarcotic, to include the following.

(1) Check each medication order against the doctor's order.

(2) Prepare the medications (check labels, accurately calculate dosages, observe proper asepsis techniques with needles and syringes).

(3) Check the patient's identification wristband to ensure positive identification before administering medications.

(4) Administer the medications. Offer each drug separately if administering more than one drug at the same time.

(5) Remain with the patient and see that the medication is taken. Never leave medications at the bedside for the patient to take later.

(6) Document the medications given as soon as possible.

f. Administer IV fluids as ordered. Maintain and monitor all IV sites. Follow SOP for infection control.

g. Participate with the health team in the patient's nutrition therapy.

h. Apply all nursing implications related to the patient diets (serving, recording intake, and food tolerance).

i. Coordinate with team leader for "take-home" wound care supplies and prescriptions for self-administration.

j. Prepare the patient and the family for disposition (transfer, return to duty, discharge). Supply the patient or family member with written instructions for:

(1) Wound care.

(2) Medications.

(3) Making outpatient appointments.

(4) An emergency, including the phone numbers for doctors and/or clinics.

k. Document the patient's disposition in the nurse's notes in accordance with unit SOP.

## 8-25. CLOSING

Surgical intervention often alters physical appearance and normal physiological functions and may threaten the patients psychological security. Any or all of these may lead to alterations in the patient's self-concept and body image. Some surgical patients react to the loss of a body part as to a death. Be aware of the patient's needs and establish interventions that will support his strengths and effective coping skills. The nursing process is used throughout the perioperative period to provide the patient with individualized care and the knowledge and ability for self-care following disposition.

*Continue with Exercises*

## EXERCISE, LESSON 8

**INSTRUCTIONS:** To complete this exercise, circle the letter of the response that best answers the question or completes the statement or write the answer in the space provided. After you have completed the all of the exercises, turn to "Solutions to Exercises" at the end of this lesson and check your answers. If you have responded to any of the exercises incorrectly, reread the material referenced after the answer.

1. ________________________ refers to the total span of surgical intervention.

2. The ________________________ phase of the surgical experience begins with the decision that surgical intervention is necessary and ends when the patient is transferred to the operating room table.

3. The ________________________ phase of the surgical experience is the period during which the patient is undergoing surgery.

4. The ________________________ phase of the surgical experience lasts from the patient's admission to the recovery room through his complete recovery from surgery.

5. Based on the degree of risk, surgery is classified as ____________ or __________.

6. ___________________ surgery is necessary, but scheduled at the convenience of the patient and the health care provider.

7. ___________________ surgery carries a high degree of risk and has the potential of postoperative complications.

8. ___________________ is the descriptor used when the purpose of a surgical procedure is to remove a diseased organ or structure.

9. When surgical intervention is to relieve pain, the purpose is described as ___________________.

10. DD Form 1924, ________________________________ has a space to document all preoperative nursing measures.

11. SF 522 ____________________________________________

____________________________________________

is a legal document, which satisfies the requirement for informed consent.

12. List five nursing implications related to the preoperative preparation of a patient.

____________________________________________

____________________________________________

____________________________________________

____________________________________________

____________________________________________

13. The key members of the surgical team are:

____________________________________________

____________________________________________

____________________________________________

____________________________________________

14. The ________________________ must have extensive knowledge of all surgical instruments and how they are used, because this member of the surgical team assists the surgeon by preparing the set-up and passing instruments.

15. The ________________________ is the liaison between scrubbed personnel in the operating room and those outside.

16. The ________________________________ is responsible for continuous monitoring of the patient's physiologic status to include oxygen exchange, systemic circulation, neurologic status, and vital signs.

17. Three major classifications of anesthetic agents are________________, ____________________, and ______________________.

18. General anesthesia produces:

______________________________________________________

______________________________________________________

______________________________________________________

______________________________________________________

19. _______________ anesthesia results in analgesia and loss of reflexes

20. _______________ anesthesia produces loss of sensation in a small area of tissue.

**SPECIAL INSTRUCTIONS FOR EXERCISES 21 THROUGH 25.** Certain drugs increase surgical risks. For exercise items 21 to 25, match the potential risk in Column I with the appropriate drug category in Column II.

| Column I | Column II |
| --- | --- |
| 21. ___ May increase the hypotensive effect of the anesthetic agent, thus contributing to shock. | a. Antibiotics in the mycine group. |
| 22. ___ May precipitate hemorrhage. | b. Anticoagulants |
| 23. ___ May cause respiratory paralysis when combined with certain muscle relaxants used during surgery. | c. Diuretics |
| 24. ___ Abrupt withdrawal may cause cardio-vascular collapse in long-term users. | d. Tranquilizers |
| 25. ___ May cause electrolyte imbalances resulting in respiratory depression from the anesthesia. | e. Adrenal steroids. |

26. Because some medications interact adversely with other medications and with anesthetic agents, preoperative assessment should include ________________ ________________________________________________.

27. General nursing goals of care for a patient in the recovery room are:

________________________________________________

________________________________________________

________________________________________________

________________________________________________

28. The most common recovery room emergency is ____________________________.

29. Respiratory status is assessed by monitoring the patient's ____________________, ____________________, and ________________________ and by observing ______________________________.

30. List four nursing implications related to the prevention of respiratory distress.

________________________________________________

________________________________________________

________________________________________________

________________________________________________

31. Four common signs and symptoms of hypovolemic shock are:

________________________________________________

________________________________________________

________________________________________________

________________________________________________

32. Nursing implications related to detection of pending hypovolemic shock include inspection of the surgical dressing. The nurse should also inspect ___________ ______________________________________________ for signs of bleeding.

33. Nursing implications related to general patient care in the recovery room include observation and documentation of______________________________________, which returns in reverse order.

34. The patient who has had a spinal anesthetic should be kept in a supine position for ____________ to _____________ hours.

35. Postoperative patient care includes receiving the patient on the nursing unit and making an initial assessment which includes:

___________________________________________________________

___________________________________________________________

___________________________________________________________

___________________________________________________________

___________________________________________________________

___________________________________________________________

___________________________________________________________

___________________________________________________________

36. Pulmonary efficiency is reduced by the effects of anesthesia on the respiratory system, increasing the possibility of _______________________________.

37. Anesthesia slows or stops the peristaltic action of the intestines resulting in ______________________________, ______________________________ .and ______________________________. Anesthesia may also cause _____________ and ______________________________resulting in a fluid imbalance.

38. Wounds heal by one of three processes: primary intention, secondary intention, or tertiary intention. ________________________________________ is healing of an open wound where there has been a significant loss of tissue.

**SPECIAL INSTRUCTIONS FOR EXERCISES 39 THROUGH 41.** Match the signs and symptoms described in Column I with the appropriate wound complications in Column II.

| Column I | Column II |
|---|---|
| 39. ___ A separation of wound edges with the protrusion of organs through the incision. | a. Wound infection |
| 40. ___ The wound edges are approximated but the wound is swollen, reddened, and feels hot. | b. Dehiscence |
| 41. ___ The wound edges are separated without protrusion of organs. | c. Evisceration |

42. Which of the following is NOT true of a Penrose drain?

a. It is made of flexible, soft rubber and causes little tissue reaction.

b. It has a reservoir to maintain constant low suction.

c. It acts by drawing any pus or fluid along its surfaces through the incision or a stab wound adjacent to the main incision.

d. The tube is pulled out and shortened 1 to 2 inches each day until it falls out.

43. Thrombophlebitis and emboli are potential complications of surgery. To prevent thrombophlebitis, instruct the patient to ______________________________ while on bed rest.

44. There are two methods of caring for wounds: the _________________ method in which no dressing is used to cover the wound and the _________________ method in which a dressing is applied.

45. Advantages of using a dressing to cover a wound are:

_______________________________________________

_______________________________________________

_______________________________________________

46. Carelessness in observing medical and surgical asepsis when changing dressings is the most common cause of ________________________________.

47. When preparing the patient and family for disposition, you should supply them with written instructions for:

_______________________________________________

_______________________________________________

_______________________________________________

_______________________________________________

***Check Your Answers on Next Page***

## SOLUTIONS TO EXERCISE, LESSON 8

1. Perioperative. (para 8-1a)

2. Preoperative (para 8-1b(1))

3. Intraoperative (para 8-1b(2))

4. Postoperative (para 8-1b(3))

5. Major; minor. (para 8-2a)

6. Elective. (para 8-2a)

7. Major. (para 8-2a(2))

8. Ablative. (para 8-2b(1))

9. Palliative. (para 8-2b(5))

10. Surgical Check List. (para 8-3b(1))

11. Request for Administration of Anesthesia and for Performance of Operations and Other Procedures. (para 8-3b(2))

12. Any five of the following.
    Assist the patient with personal hygiene and related preoperative care.
    Provide information concerning surgery.
    Provide preoperative morning care.
    Remove prostheses.
    Record vital signs.
    Recheck the accuracy of DD Form 1924.
    Administer preoperative medications.
    Assist the operating room technician. (paras 8-4a--e)

13. The surgeon.
    The anesthesiologist or anesthetist.
    The scrub nurse or scrub assistant.
    The circulating nurse. (paras 8-6b--e)

14. Scrub nurse/assistant. (para 8-6d)

15. Circulating nurse. (para 8-6e)

16. Anesthesiologist/anesthetist. (para 8-6c(4))

17. General; regional; local. (para 8-7a)

18. Narcosis.
Analgesia.
Lose of reflexes.
Relaxation. (para 8-8a)

19. Regional. (para 8-8a)

20. Local. (para 8-8a)

21. d (para 8-8d(2))

22. b (para 8-8d(2))

23. a (para 8-8d(2))

24. e (para 8-8d(2))

25. c (para 8-8d(2))

26. A thorough medication history. (para 8□8d(1))

27. To support the patient through his state of dependence to independence.
To relieve the patient's discomfort.
Early detection of complications.
Prevention of complications. (paras 8-10a(1)--(4))

28. Respiratory distress. (para 8-11a)

29. Respiratory rate; rhythm; depth; skin color. (para 8-12a)

30. Any four of the following.
Monitor respiratory status.
Report labored respirations to the supervisor.
Report shallow, rapid respirations to the supervisor.
Maintain a patent airway.
Maintain the patient in a position to facilitate lung expansion.
Administer oxygen as ordered.
Prevent aspiration of vomitus.
Suction the patient as ordered. (para 8-12a--h)

31. Any four of the following.
    Hypotension.
    Cold, clammy skin.
    A weak, thready, and rapid pulse.
    Deep, rapid respirations.
    Decreased urine output.
    Thirst.
    Apprehension.
    Restlessness. (para 8-13a)

32. The bedding beneath the patient. (para 8-14a)

33. Level of consciousness. (para 8-15b(3))

34. Six; eight. (para 8-15b(5))

35. Position and safety.
    Vital signs.
    Level of consciousness.
    Intravenous fluids.
    Wound.
    Drains and tubes.
    Skin color and temperature.
    Comfort. (paras 8-16b(1)--(7))

36. Pneumonia. (para 8-17a(1))

37. Constipation, abdominal distention, flatulence; nausea, vomiting. (para 8-17a(4))

38. Secondary intention. (para 8-20a(2))

39. c (para 8-19a(3))

40. a (para 8-19a(1))

41. b (para 8-19a(2))

42. b (para 8-22b)

43. Exercise the legs while on bedrest. (para 8-23b)

44. Open; closed. (para 8-23e(1))

45. Dressings absorb drainage.
Dressings protect the wound from injury and contamination.
Dressings provide physical, psychological, and aesthetic comfort for the patient.
(para 8-23e(1))

46. Nosocomial infections. (8-23e(2))

47. Wound care.
Medications.
Making outpatient appointments.
An emergency, including the phone numbers for the doctor and/or clinic.
(para 8-24i)

***End of Lesson 8***

Printed in Dunstable, United Kingdom

91338753R00219